Healthcare Simulation
at a Glance

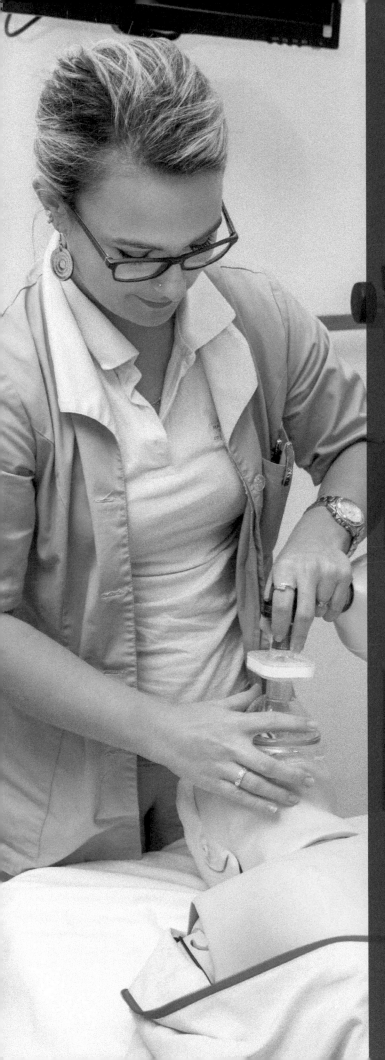

Healthcare Simulation at a Glance

Edited by

Kirsty Forrest
Professor of Medical Education and Research,
Dean of Medicine, Faculty of Health Sciences
and Medicine, Bond University, Gold Coast,
Australia

Judy McKimm
Professor of Medical Education and Director
of Strategic Educational Development, Swansea
University Medical School, Swansea, UK
Visiting Professor, King Saud University, Riyadh,
Kingdom of Saudi Arabia

WILEY Blackwell

This edition first published 2019
© 2019 John Wiley & Sons Ltd.

The right of Kirsty Forrest and Judy McKimm to be identified as the authors of the editorial material in this work has been asserted in accordance with law.

Registered Offices:
John Wiley & Sons, Inc., 111 River Street, Hoboken, NJ 07030, USA
John Wiley & Sons Ltd, The Atrium, Southern Gate, Chichester,
West Sussex, PO19 8SQ, UK

Editorial Office
9600 Garsington Road, Oxford, OX4 2DQ, UK

For details of our global editorial offices, customer services, and more information about Wiley products visit us at www.wiley.com.

Wiley also publishes its books in a variety of electronic formats and by print-on-demand. Some content that appears in standard print versions of this book may not be available in other formats.

Limit of Liability/Disclaimer of Warranty
The contents of this work are intended to further general scientific research, understanding, and discussion only and are not intended and should not be relied upon as recommending or promoting scientific method, diagnosis, or treatment by physicians for any particular patient. In view of ongoing research, equipment modifications, changes in governmental regulations, and the constant flow of information relating to the use of medicines, equipment, and devices, the reader is urged to review and evaluate the information provided in the package insert or instructions for each medicine, equipment, or device for, among other things, any changes in the instructions or indication of usage and for added warnings and precautions. While the publisher and authors have used their best efforts in preparing this work, they make no representations or warranties with respect to the accuracy or completeness of the contents of this work and specifically disclaim all warranties, including without limitation any implied warranties of merchantability or fitness for a particular purpose. No warranty may be created or extended by sales representatives, written sales materials or promotional statements for this work. The fact that an organization, website, or product is referred to in this work as a citation and/or potential source of further information does not mean that the publisher and authors endorse the information or services the organization, website, or product may provide or recommendations it may make. This work is sold with the understanding that the publisher is not engaged in rendering professional services. The advice and strategies contained herein may not be suitable for your situation. You should consult with a specialist where appropriate. Further, readers should be aware that websites listed in this work may have changed or disappeared between when this work was written and when it is read. Neither the publisher nor authors shall be liable for any loss of profit or any other commercial damages, including but not limited to special, incidental, consequential, or other damages.

Library of Congress Cataloging-in-Publication Data
Names: Forrest, Kirsty, editor. | McKimm, Judy, editor.
Title: Healthcare simulation at a glance / edited by Kirsty Forrest, Judy McKimm.
Description: Hoboken, NJ : Wiley-Blackwell, 2019. | Series: At a glance
  series | Includes bibliographical references and index. |
Identifiers: LCCN 2019017159 (print) | LCCN 2019018355 (ebook) | ISBN
  9781118871829 (Adobe PDF) | ISBN 9781118871836 (ePub) | ISBN 9781118871843
  (paperback)
Subjects: | MESH: Education, Medical--methods | Simulation Training | Handbook
Classification: LCC R837.S55 (ebook) | LCC R837.S55 (print) | NLM W 49 | DDC
  610.1/1--dc23
LC record available at https://lccn.loc.gov/2019017159

Cover image: © choja / Getty Images
Cover design by Wiley

Set in Minion Pro 9.5/11.5 by Aptara
Printed by CPI Group (UK) Ltd, Croydon CR0 4YY

10 9 8 7 6 5 4 3 2 1

Contents

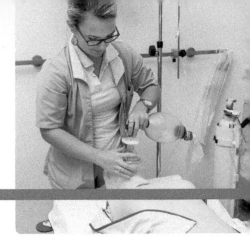

Part 5 Developing your practice 75

Contributors

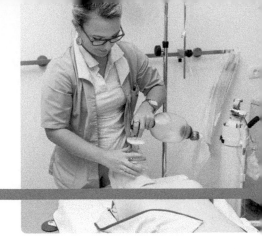

Kash Akhtar Chapter 4
Senior Clinical Academic Lecturer, Barts and the London School of Medicine and Dentistry, QMUL and Consultant Trauma and Orthopaedic Surgeon, Barts Health NHS Trust, London, UK

Pamela Andreatta Chapter 6
Professor, University of Central Florida, Orlando, Florida, USA

Margaret Bearman Chapters 7, 10
Associate Professor, Centre for Research in Assessment and Digital Learning (CRADLE), Deakin University, Australia

Fernando Bello Chapters 17, 18
Professor of Surgical Computing and Simulation Science, Imperial College, London, UK

Laurence Boss Chapter 28
Consultant Anaesthetist, Guy's and St Thomas' Hospitals NHS Foundation Trust, London, UK

Victoria Brazil Chapters 5, 19
Professor of Emergency Medicine, Bond University, Australia

Arunangsu Chatterjee Chapter 16
Associate Professor, Director of Technology Enhanced Learning and Distance Learning, Plymouth University Peninsula Schools of Medicine and Dentistry, Plymouth, UK

Faiza Chowdhury Chapters 13, 14, 20, 21
Clinical Research Fellow, Imperial College, London, UK

Kirsty Forrest Chapters 2, 24, 30, 34
Professor of Medical Education and Research, Dean of Medicine, Faculty of Health Sciences and Medicine, Bond University, Gold Coast, Australia

Andi Fox-Hiley Chapter 11
Health Care Education Advisor, Leeds Teaching Hospitals, Leeds, UK

Thomas Gale Chapters 25, 26, 29
Clinical Associate Professor, Director of Clinical Skills and Simulation, Plymouth University Peninsula Schools of Medicine and Dentistry, Plymouth, UK

Jivendra Gosai Chapter 14
Consultant Cardiologist, Bradford Royal Infirmary, Bradford, UK

Mark Hellaby Chapters 1, 3, 15
North West Simulation Education Network Manager, NHS Health Education England, London, UK

Roger Kneebone Chapters 17, 18
Professor of Surgical Education and Engagement Science, Imperial College, London, UK

Andy Kordowicz Chapters 20, 21
Consultant Vascular Surgeon, York Hospitals NHS Foundation Trust, York, UK

Al May Chapter 28
Associate Director and Faculty Development Lead, Scottish Centre for Simulation and Clinical Human Factors, Larburt, UK

Michelle McKenzie Smith Chapter 8
Clinical Skills, Simulation, Resuscitation and Manual Handling Manager, Doncaster and Bassetlaw Teaching Hospitals NHS Trust, Doncaster, UK

Judy McKimm Chapters 24, 32, 33
Professor of Medical Education and Director of Strategic Educational Development, Swansea University Medical School, Swansea, UK

Nancy McNaughton Chapter 31
Director, Centre for Learning, Innovation and Simulation, Michener Institute of Education at UHN, Toronto, Ontario

Maggie Meeks Chapter 27
Clinical Education Advisor and Neonatal Paediatrician, University of Otago, Otago, New Zealand

Fidelity is commonly used to mean how life-like or authentic a simulation or piece of equipment is, but this meaning of the term is often contested in healthcare simulation.

The term fidelity was initially used to describe aircraft simulation where, historically, transposing the instruments and technology from the real cockpit to a simulated cockpit allowed a recreation of the area with a high degree of fidelity. One of the main issues around the term fidelity in healthcare simulation is that we ultimately treat and interact with humans not technology, therefore it is virtually impossible to recreate all elements of the simulation faithfully and there will always be some disconnect. The traditional view of fidelity is that the various elements that comprise a simulation, cumulatively form its overall fidelity. There has been considerable discussion about the construct of fidelity, the elements and the areas covered, and a lack of a uniformly agreed definition or descriptor.

Often fidelity is described as comprising the manikin (equipment) fidelity, environmental fidelity and psychological fidelity, although task fidelity, physical fidelity and functional fidelity have also been described (Rehmann et al., 1995). The manikin fidelity element is further subdivided into low, medium and high fidelity depending on the degree to which the manikin mimics a real patient.

Hamstra et al. (2014), however, suggest that the focus should not just be on how real the manikin looks but also on how well the simulation process engages with the learners, transfers the learning and suspends disbelief: all which affect educational effectiveness.

Simulation vs. manikin fidelity

Another issue with the term fidelity is confusion around the blurring of distinction between high, medium and low simulation fidelity and high, medium and low manikin fidelity. All too often manikin fidelity is equated with the overall simulation fidelity, assuming high fidelity manikin = high fidelity scenario and low fidelity manikin = low fidelity scenario. However, this does not take into account all the other fidelity elements that impact on the learning experience. For example, Figure 3.1 shows a medium fidelity manikin in the low fidelity setting of a classroom. This cannot be presumed to be a medium fidelity simulation just because the manikin is medium fidelity.

In team training (Figure 3.2), manikin fidelity may be a small component of the overall simulation fidelity because the real focus is on team working and communication. This helps explain why substituting a much lower fidelity manikin seems to do very little to the overall simulation fidelity. When designing simulation activities, therefore, educators need to consider carefully how realistic, authentic or high fidelity each of the components needs to be. In some simulations (e.g. an OSCE (objective structured clinical examination) station) it might be beneficial to use a simulated patient rather than a manikin, whereas in others a rudimentary, low fidelity piece of equipment will perform just as well.

Figure 3.3 demonstrates a low (manikin) fidelity tracheostomy part task trainer used for a simulation in an intensive care unit (ICU). The manikin, together with a monitor emulator used to simulate a realistic critical care monitor, is used in a dislodged tracheostomy scenario. This takes part in the actual clinical area with the real clinical team (ultimate environmental fidelity). In this setting, the learners experience psychological stressors from the tone of the pulse oximeter on the desaturated 'patient' as in 'real' life. Therefore, although we are using a low fidelity manikin, it is clear that this is a high fidelity simulation. Figure 3.4 demonstrates the appropriate use of a low fidelity injection trainer whereas Figure 3.5 shows that for other skills this trainer would not be as appropriate. Box 3.1 includes some basic top tips.

Hamstra and colleagues (2014) further critiqued the use of the term manikin fidelity by pointing out that the manikin's fidelity is actually dynamic depending on the particular learning outcomes and the manikin used. So whilst the low fidelity manikin in the ICU scenario was entirely appropriate and provided a high fidelity simulation, it could be argued that in this simulation it was actually a high fidelity manikin.

In theory, this argument can be extended to other fidelity elements. For instance, whilst environmental fidelity appears more important than equipment in the ICU scenario, it may be less so for a surgeon practising using a surgical skills' simulator.

Fidelity vs. learning outcomes

There is no evidence that increasing fidelity improves the level of learning outcomes or engagement, and the real disadvantage of chasing higher levels of overall fidelity is that costs increase. The primary aim of educators is to provide a safe learning environment for learners. This is partly achieved by leaners recognising that this is a simulation, designed so that they can make mistakes and not harm a real patient. This encourages learners to participate in simulation activities and it is possible that by making the simulation 'too real', its educational effectiveness is actually reduced.

The solution?

If the term fidelity causes so much confusion what should we do? Hamstra et al. (2014) suggest replacing the phrase 'manikin fidelity' with the terms: 'physical resemblance' and 'functional task alignment'. Another suggestion is to focus on 'realism' rather than fidelity. However, simulation educators need to be aware that this issue is still under debate and the confusion about the term fidelity will probably remain for some time.

Research in healthcare simulation

Practice points

- Research in healthcare should utilise fundamental principles of research, including educational approaches
- Research designs can include quantitative, qualitative or mixed research methodologies
- Evaluation of the impact of simulation education and its translation into clinical care is an imperative

Figure 4.1 The Kirkpatrick framework of evaluation applied to simulation research.

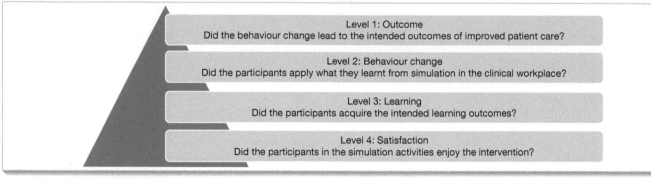

Level 1: Outcome
Did the behaviour change lead to the intended outcomes of improved patient care?

Level 2: Behaviour change
Did the participants apply what they learnt from simulation in the clinical workplace?

Level 3: Learning
Did the participants acquire the intended learning outcomes?

Level 4: Satisfaction
Did the participants in the simulation activities enjoy the intervention?

Table 4.1 Contributions of medical education interventions as translational science. Source: Adapted from W. C. McGaghie, Medical education research as translational science. *Sci. Transl. Med.* **2**, 19cm8 (2010).

	Level of translational research		
	T1	**T2**	**T3**
What is increased or improved?	Knowledge, skill, attitudes and professionalism	Patient care practices	Patient outcomes
Who is the target?	Individuals and teams	Individuals and teams	Individuals and public health
Where is the setting/intervention?	Simulation lab	Clinic and bedside	Clinic and community

Box 4.1 Examples of types of quantitative research designs.

- **Descriptive research:** statistical research in order to demonstrate and describe relationships
- **Experimental research:** the testing of a hypothesis and establishing causation by manipulating independent and dependent variables in a controlled environment
- **Causal-comparative research:** used to explore and explain the differences that exist between groups of individuals by determining cause and effect
- **Correlational research:** used to explore but not explain the differences that exist between groups of individuals
- **Meta-analysis:** a statistical technique to combine results from multiple independent studies in order to test the data for significance

Box 4.2 Examples of types of qualitative research designs.

- **Grounded theory:** systematic processes used to generate a general explanation of a process, actions or interactions. The explanation emerges from the data
- **Ethnography:** where a researcher (usually an outsider) uses defined processes to describe and understand a particular setting through detailed observation
- **Action research:** centres on an alteration in practice that is analysed and evaluated, resulting in further changes. This is an empirically based spiral improvement process
- **Narrative research:** seeks to understand human behaviour through the use of text, stories, biographies, photographs and correspondence, etc.
- **Phenomenology:** attempts to uncover people's perceptions, perspectives and understandings of a particular situation (or phenomenon). It uses interviews, observations, diaries, drawings, etc.

Box 4.3 Concepts of validity in quantitative research.

- **Face validity:** the acceptability of a tool
- **Construct validity:** the ability of a tool to differentiate between subjects of varying expertise and ability
- **Content validity:** a judgement of the appropriateness of a tool as determined by experts in the field
- **Concurrent validity:** the correlation between performance as measured by a tool against an accepted and established form of assessment
- **Predictive validity:** the extent to which a tool predicts future performance

Box 4.4 Concepts of trustworthiness in qualitative research.

- **Triangulation:** using multiple data sources, analysers, time periods and sites to confirm findings
- **Theoretical sampling strategies:** the confirmation of theories developed to describe trends seen in data
- **Respondent validation:** the collection of feedback from participants about the accuracy of data they have provided and the interpretation of that data by researchers
- **Promoting participant honesty:** ensuring confidentiality, opportunities to withdraw from the study
- **Iterative questioning:** returning to similar concepts within an interview through rephrasing of questions
- **Check for researcher effects:** analysing the data for potential causes of bias by researchers (reflexivity)
- **Peer review:** discussing processes and results regularly with other researchers through the period of the research

Healthcare Simulation at a Glance. First Edition. Kirsty Forrest and Judy McKimm. © 2019 John Wiley & Sons, Ltd.
Published 2019 by John Wiley & Sons, Ltd.

Healthcare simulation research includes studies *about* simulation (as an educational method) and studies that *use* simulation to investigate other things (Gaba, 2015). Examples include research into the role of simulation for the acquisition of psychomotor skills, in developing teamwork skills and in improving patient outcomes. Robust research is essential to advance the science and practice of healthcare simulation. Researchers use conventional research methods from the sciences and social sciences; the selection of method depends on the research question.

A thorough literature review is key to ensuring access to the latest knowledge and evidence, and helps to identify areas of uncertainty ripe for study. Depending on the research aim and question, the most appropriate research methods should be used to obtain data for analysis. These results form the basis of a discussion and conclusion that addresses the research question posed.

Kirkpatrick's (1994) framework to evaluate (and research) the impact of (simulation) training is commonly used (Figure 4.1). Translational patient outcomes have been described for healthcare simulation (McGaghie, 2010; McGaghie et al., 2011a). Most studies are at the level of T1, demonstrating changes in the 'educational laboratory', with some studies at T2, demonstrating 'improved downstream patient care', and very few at T3, demonstrating changes in patient and public health (Table 4.1) (McGaghie et al., 2011a).

Ethics of simulation-based research

Institutional or national ethics committee approval must be obtained before commencing any simulation research. Participants are usually asked to provide informed consent. Although in this type of research it is unlikely that anyone will be harmed, any possible physical or psychological effects need to be considered. For example, participants may feel coerced to take part or under pressure to produce the 'right' result as they may work in the same department as, or be students of, those performing the research. Respecting confidentiality, highlighting the voluntary nature of research and the ability to withdraw without disadvantage is important. Researchers must act with probity and all conflicts of interest must be declared at the outset.

Research design

An appropriate research design ensures that studies are robust and reproducible. These will also safeguard researchers and participants by enforcing compliance to pre-approved research protocols. Boxes 4.1 and 4.2 summarise commonly used research designs such as *quantitative* or *qualitative* or a combination, called mixed methods. Quantitative research usually tries to answer 'who' or 'what' questions while qualitative research looks for answers to 'why' and 'how' questions.

Quantitative methods

For research to be robust it is imperative to have a well-defined experimental design and to obtain reliable data for statistical analysis. The gold standard is the randomised, controlled, double-blinded study but this is not always possible in simulation research as it can be difficult to blind participants. Designing a study begins by performing a power calculation in order to ensure enough participants are recruited to adequately demonstrate any significance. Appropriate randomisation must be utilised as well as control subjects if possible. It is important to eliminate confounding factors or sources of bias.

Virtual reality simulators provide objective technical metrics appropriate for quantitative analysis. However, proxy tools can be used when researching factors such as human behaviour and performance. These allow more abstract skills to be observed and measured to produce numerical data. Global rating scales are used to assess psychomotor skills and domains such as decision making and interpersonal communication. However, tools must first be shown to be valid and reliable. Many types of validity exist which reflect different aspects that work synergistically to address whether a tool is an accurate measure of the task under review (Box 4.3).

The reliability of a tool is a measure of its consistency in providing the same results on repeated testing. This is key if it is to be widely used for assessing performance and if benchmarking and comparison of results is desired. This can be determined statistically by calculating the test–retest coefficient, the internal consistency coefficient and intra- and inter-rater reliability. These last two are particularly relevant when using more subjective assessments such as global rating scales. In 2016 reporting guidelines were published for simulation-based education interventions (Cheng et al., 2016).

Qualitative methods

Qualitative research is used when researchers seek answers to questions or explanations of phenomena using predefined processes. It usually seeks to understand a problem, issue or phenomenon in a particular context. Commonly used methods include observations, in-depth interviews and focus groups (Box 4.2). Different techniques are used to systematically analyse data. Transcripts are made of audio-recorded data enabling analysis of text. Commonly, codes are identified and then clustered into themes. Further analysis seeks relationships between themes. Sample sizes are usually smaller than in quantitative research. Qualitative researchers practice reflexivity, acknowledging their position and impact on the process and outcomes of research (Creswell, 2011). Qualitative researchers are less concerned with validity than quantitative researchers but, instead, refer to concepts of trustworthiness (Box 4.4) (Guba, 1981; Shenton, 2004).

Summary

Conducting research in healthcare simulation draws on the principles of research. Many of the common methodological flaws can be minimised through adhering to a well-structured experimental design. A thorough literature review will ensure a breadth of knowledge about the field of study, that work is not repeated and that previous errors can be avoided. Performing a statistical power analysis at the outset will ensure that a study is not underpowered and appropriate randomisation should result in an equal distribution of confounding factors. Using the correct research methodology is key to achieving a robust study. Valid and reliable measures must be used for data collection to permit accurate analysis and conclusions. These factors will combine to produce studies that advance knowledge within simulation and help to further develop the specialty.

5 The evidence base for simulation education

Practice points

- Effective simulation education has similar characteristics to other effective educational encounters
- There is growing evidence for procedural and teamwork skills acquisition using simulation-based education
- More evidence is needed to show whether simulation education improves patient outcomes

Figure 5.1 Teamwork training.

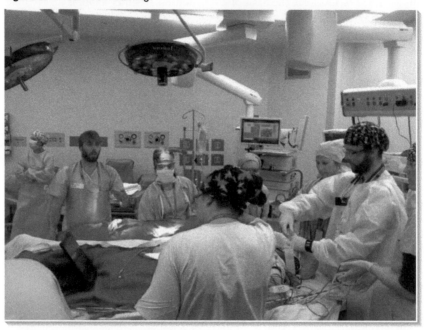

Box 5.1 Features and uses of high-fidelity medical simulations that lead to effective learning: a BEME systematic review. Source: Adapted from Issenberg et al., 2005.

- Providing feedback
- Repetitive practice
- Curriculum integration
- Range of difficulty levels
- Multiple learning strategies
- Capturing clinical variation
- Controlled (safe) environment
- Individualised learning
- Defined outcomes
- Simulator validity (i.e. realism)

Box 5.2 Nine elements of deliberate practice (DP). Source: Adapted from McGaghie, Siddall et al., 2009.

- Highly motivated learners with good concentration who address ...
- Well-defined learning objectives or tasks at an ...
- Appropriate level of difficulty with ...
- Focused, repetitive practice that yields ...
- Rigorous, reliable measurements that provide ...
- Informative feedback from educational sources (e.g. simulators, teachers) that Promote ...
- Monitoring, error correction, and more deliberate practice that enable ...
- Evaluation and performance that may reach a mastery standard where learning time may vary but expected minimal outcomes are identical and allows ...
- Advancement to the next task or unit

Box 5.3 Case study – evidence for patient outcomes.

An institution decides to improve its 'time to CT' performance for paediatric head injury patients, aware that this is a time critical condition. Baseline data are collected on current performance. An in situ programme of simulated scenarios is designed and delivered over a 6-month period – involving the emergency department team, neurosurgeons and medical imaging staff. There is a debriefing after each simulation, focused on process improvements. After the 6-month programme, performance is re-measured and found to be significantly improved

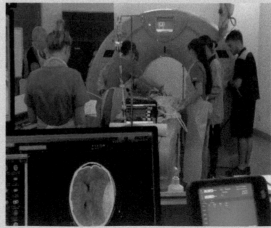

Healthcare Simulation at a Glance. First Edition. Kirsty Forrest and Judy McKimm. © 2019 John Wiley & Sons, Ltd.
Published 2019 by John Wiley & Sons, Ltd.

As an emerging and resource-intensive teaching modality, simulation-based [medical] education (SB[M]E) has been scrutinised for 'evidence' of effectiveness. Finding this evidence is first hampered by the difficulty of defining 'effectiveness'. The outcomes for simulation training are broad, ranging from discrete procedural skills, complex teamwork and leadership behaviours to patient-based outcomes. Randomised, controlled trials (the gold standard) are rarely performed in healthcare education and are arguably a poor methodology for finding evidence for SBE.

Evidence for what?

Instead of asking 'Does simulation work?', a more useful approach is to examine the features that make SBE effective for the specific content or aim intended. Issenberg and colleagues (2005) conducted a best evidence in medical education (BEME) systematic review asking this question, and reviewed a focused set of 109 studies. The results indicated that the most important features of SBME for effectiveness were similar to those for almost any effective teaching method (Box 5.1).

Procedural skills

McGaghie and colleagues (2011b) undertook a comparative review of SBME versus traditional clinical education for the focused outcome of skills acquisition, and found a large and quantifiable effect size. However, this study compared SBME used for a specific method (i.e. deliberate practice, Box 5.2) (McGaghie et al., 2009), not just the use of simulation or manikins/part task trainers per se.

Multiple studies have shown quantifiable improvements in learners' procedural skills because of SBME. Surgical simulators and part task trainers can offer a high physical resemblance to real procedural skill situations. Learning curves and task analysis for single operator procedures are often more easily quantified than more complex behavioural skills. Dawe et al. (2014) concluded that a high 'transferability' of skills was acquired on simulator-based training compared with patient-based training for endoscopy and laparoscopic cholecystectomy.

Teamwork skills

Increasing recognition of teamwork as vital for optimal healthcare outcomes and patient safety has resulted in many publications examining strategies for optimal team training (Figure 5.1).

Weaver et al. (2014) undertook a literature review, identifying 90–100 publications per year on healthcare teamwork training. The review found that there were many effective modalities for team training, including classroom and simulation-based interventions. Several studies showed significant improvement in team functioning following simulation-based team training. In addition, simulation has been used for the development and validation of robust measures of team function, to facilitate structured observation and feedback, and to allow benchmarking.

Patient outcomes

Evaluation of SBME (or any health professions' education) is rarely undertaken at the level of patient outcomes.

McGaghie et al. (2011a) conducted a qualitative synthesis of SBME translational science research (TSR), looking at how SBME addresses healthcare delivery yielding measurable improvement in the health of individuals and society (see Table 4.1). Fifteen research reports were summarised and conclusions drawn that:

> … translational science research outcomes are more likely when SBME interventions are embedded in rigorous educational and health services research programs that are thematic, sustained, and cumulative. (McGaghie et al., 2011a)

Hence SBME can improve health service level outcome if it is part of the overall plan for quality improvement, and not just a 'one-off' teaching activity. See the case study in Box 5.3.

Notable examples exist where SBME directed at the level of the team or unit has improved patient outcomes. These include the following:

• Draycott et al. (2006) demonstrated statistically and clinically significant reductions in birth complications following shoulder dystocia after the implementation of a team-based SBME programme.
• Trauma team training using SBME has not only improved a variety of team performance measures, but also improved clinical outcomes – time to computed tomography (CT) scanner, time to endotracheal intubation and operating room transfer time (Capella et al., 2010).
• An implementation of a paediatric 'mock code' programme improved survival rates by approximately 50% ($P = 0.000$), significantly above the average national paediatric cardiopulmonary arrest survival rates, and correlating with the increased number of mock codes ($r = 0.87$) (Andreatta et al., 2011).

Summary

Finding evidence for SBME is elusive. However, rigorous evaluation of impact of SBME interventions should occur in the context of the aims and objectives of those programmes, and features that lead to effectiveness identified. In general, learning and evaluation strategies that result in effective healthcare education and training are also applicable to simulation-based medical education.

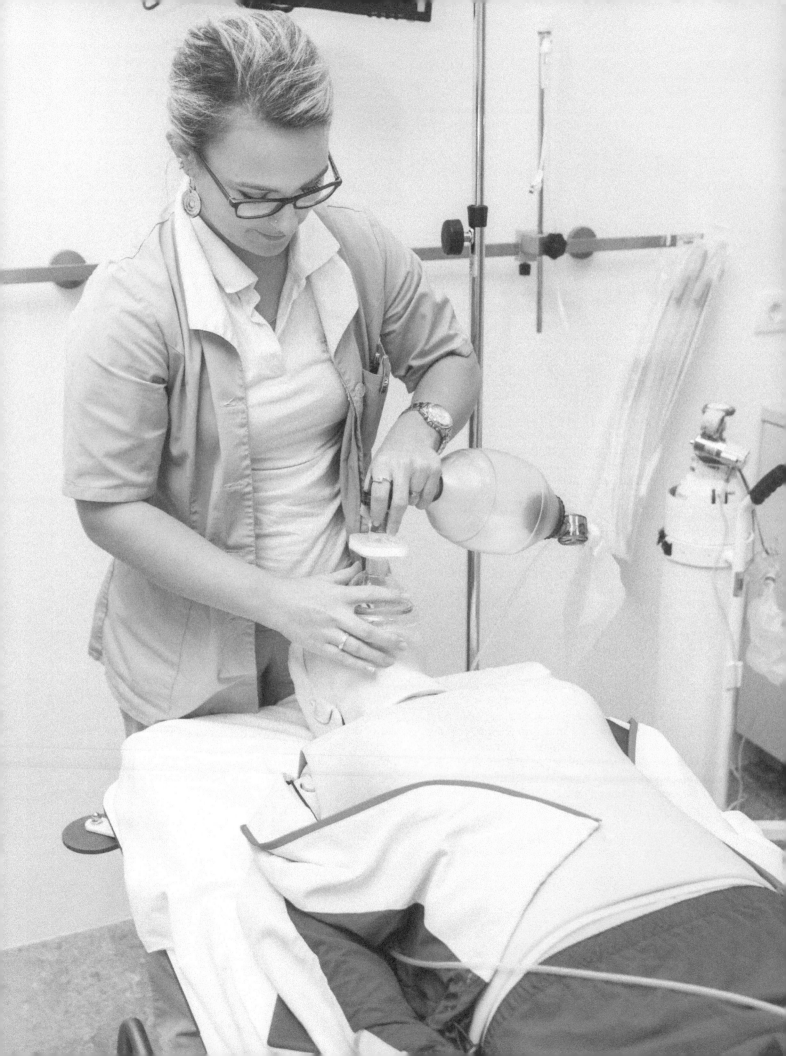

Simulation and education

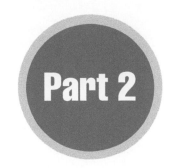
Part 2

Chapters

6 Learning theories and simulation education: 1

Practice points

- Simulation-based education provides an ideal experiential learning environment, as opportunities for reflection and experimentation are inherent in the methodology
- Simulation education is well supported by the theories of behaviourism and cognitivism
- The concepts of deliberate practice and automaticity are central to using simulation to develop motor skills

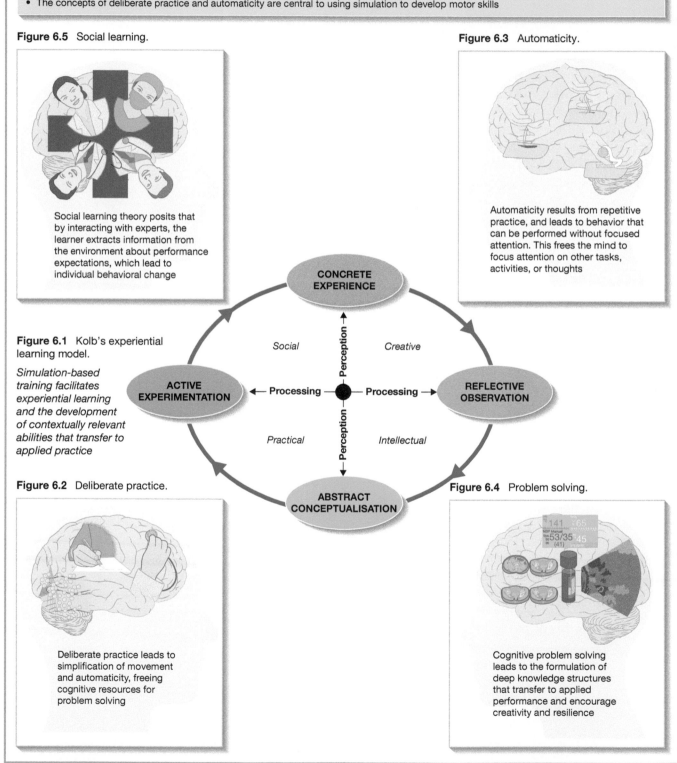

Figure 6.5 Social learning.

Social learning theory posits that by interacting with experts, the learner extracts information from the environment about performance expectations, which lead to individual behavioral change

Figure 6.3 Automaticity.

Automaticity results from repetitive practice, and leads to behavior that can be performed without focused attention. This frees the mind to focus attention on other tasks, activities, or thoughts

Figure 6.1 Kolb's experiential learning model.

Simulation-based training facilitates experiential learning and the development of contextually relevant abilities that transfer to applied practice

Figure 6.2 Deliberate practice.

Deliberate practice leads to simplification of movement and automaticity, freeing cognitive resources for problem solving

Figure 6.4 Problem solving.

Cognitive problem solving leads to the formulation of deep knowledge structures that transfer to applied performance and encourage creativity and resilience

Healthcare Simulation at a Glance. First Edition. Kirsty Forrest and Judy McKimm. © 2019 John Wiley & Sons, Ltd.
Published 2019 by John Wiley & Sons, Ltd.

Experiential learning theory

This suggests that learning is best achieved when individuals actively engage with authentic experiences in a content domain, and then reflect on those experiences to derive relevance (abstraction) they can test in other contexts. Kolb's model for this cycle expands on the constructivist foundations established by Dewey, who theorized that the successive processes of interaction, reflection and abstraction of concepts led to better understanding and retention over time (Dewey, 1933). Kolb further proposed that analytical skills were necessary for conceptualisation and that a process of active experimentation to test those abstractions was essential for acquiring expertise (Figure 6.1) (Kolb, 1984).

Historically, healthcare has used an apprenticeship model for learning wherein learners engage in direct patient care. However, this is not an ideal experiential environment because the opportunities for reflection and experimentation are limited, and concerns about patient safety are paramount. Simulation-based education (SBE) serves to ameliorate those concerns and facilitate an experiential environment in which learners and clinicians can acquire, refine and maintain their abilities in contextually relevant situations, without impacting patient or clinician safety. Further, best practices in SBE prescribe a deliberate process for reflection that furthers connections between theory and practice, the transfer of learning to other areas of professional experience, and development for individuals and teams. Reflective practice can identify strengths and areas for improvement, and an understanding of the beliefs, attitudes and values that impact performance. For clinicians who work in the ever-changing field of healthcare, reflective practice is a powerful process for assuring they provide up-to-date, high quality care (Davies, 2012).

Behaviourism and deliberate practice

Simulation-based experiential learning environments are also well supported by other theoretical foundations. These can be viewed through the integration of two primary considerations: behaviour (performance) and cognition (problem solving). Behaviourism focuses on objective observation of perceptual and motor modules of behaviour (actions) rather than the unobservable events that take place in the mind (Skinner, 1963). From a learning perspective, the process of action–response interactions within an environment leads to changes in behaviour. The more repetitions of a positive action–response interaction that can be accomplished, the more rapidly the actions will be mastered and retained by the learner. The process is known as deliberate practice, whereby learners' performance in a learning context is facilitated by expert feedback about their performance alongside expected targets (Ericsson et al., 1993). Expert feedback helps learners minimise the errors and frustration associated with trial and error processes, as well as reducing the likelihood of poor performance factors becoming habituated and therefore more difficult to remediate (Figure 6.2).

Several factors influence performance improvement, including the frequency of engagement and the effectiveness of resulting feedback. Effective feedback includes specific information about how the performance compares with the expected standards and how the learner can modify or further improve their performance. Ineffective feedback, or no feedback,

during deliberate practice may delay or be detrimental to learning. Likewise, if a learner does not practice with sufficient frequency, reinforcement will fade and acquired skills may be forgotten. The frequency of practice will depend on the activity itself (its complexity), as well as the learner's pre-existing abilities in the performance domain prior to learning the new skills. The more novice the learner or complex the performance, the more likely frequent practice over an extended period will be necessary to achieve performance objectives.

Automaticity

Automaticity results when sufficient practice leads to the ability to perform actions without thinking about them. Examples include walking, riding a bike, driving a car, knot tying, hand washing, etc. Achieving automaticity allows the performer to attend to other events in the environment while continuing to execute the automated activities without compromise because the automatic mental processes do not require significant mental resources (Bargh, 1994). Automaticity results from overlearning behaviours until they become reflexive, thereby allowing learners to devote attention to other important tasks, problem solving or creative improvisation. The cognitive processes associated with innovation and creativity requires a degree of automaticity to facilitate the reorganisation of reflexive behaviours into something novel or unique (Figure 6.3).

Cognitivism

Cognitivism refers to covert processes, or acts of mind, such as processing perceptions, memory retrieval and problem solving (Vygotsky, 2003). Goal-related activities always require some degree of problem solving to determine how to move – step by step – from the existing state to the goal state. Mature, sophisticated problem solving requires domain-specific expertise that facilitates identifying potential problems in advance to avoid problems and inefficiencies on the way to goal attainment.

It can take an expert thousands of hours to develop their ability to easily recognise and remember significant patterns. An expert knows thousands of domain-specific patterns and rules, but also knows when to *break* those rules, which is almost as important as knowing the rules themselves (Pretz et al., 2003). Experts can recognise rare events in a domain as well as events that appear to be one thing but may actually be another. Similarly, experts are adept at selecting the best option from available alternatives. The acquisition and maintenance of expertise is an ongoing process for healthcare providers, and includes assemblage of contextually based knowledge of the healthcare environment itself (Figure 6.4).

Social learning theory

This theory posits a reciprocal relationship between an individual's behaviour and their social and physical environment, such that each influences the other. Through observation and feedback, the learner extracts information from the environment about performance expectations (Bandura, 1977). Simulation-based environments that adequately model the real healthcare environment will imbue learners with more transferrable expertise than those with less contextual fidelity (Figure 6.5).

7 Learning theories and simulation education: 2

Practice points

- Constructivism, social cognitive theory, situated learning theory and activity theory come from different traditions, but all recognise the role of context in learning
- Simulation designs and associated debriefings can optimise opportunities for learners to regulate their own cognitive and emotional response to challenges

Box 7.1 Constructivism. Source: Biggs (1996). Reproduced with permission of Springer.

"...a consensus [view of constructivism] would be that **learners arrive at meaning** by **actively selecting**, and **cumulatively constructing**, their own knowledge, through both **individual and social activity**. The learner brings an **accumulation of assumptions, motives, intentions, and previous knowledge** ...the **centrality of the learner** is given."

Box 7.2 Social cognitive theory.

"The capacity to **exercise control** over the **nature and quality of one's life** is the essence of humanness.... **Personal agency** operates within a **broad network** of sociostructural influences. In these agentic transactions, **people are producers as well as products of social systems**."

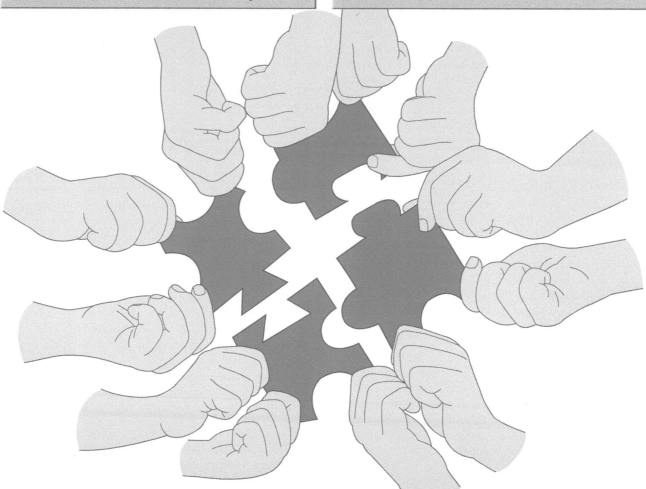

Box 7.3 Situated learning. Source: Brown et al. (1989). Reproduced with permission of SAGE.

"The activity in which **knowledge is developed and deployed**, it is now argued, is **not separable** from or ancillary to **learning and cognition**. Nor is it neutral. Rather, it is **an integral part of what is learned**. Situations might be said to **co-produce knowledge through activity**."

Box 7.4 Activity theory. Source: Fenwick et al. (2011). Reproduced with permission of Routledge.

"The **concept of activity** is premised on an understanding of **learning, human development and education**, as a matter of **what, why and how people do things together**, either **cooperatively** or **conflictually**, over time."

Constructivism, social cognitive theory, situated learning theory and activity theory come from different traditions, but all recognise the role of context in learning and can be applied to simulation-based education (SBE).

Constructivism

Constructivism is strongly aligned with notions of 'learner-centred education'. Some consider constructivism more of an orientation towards learning than a theory per se (Dennick, 2012). Its core tenet is that learning is not about receiving information but about active participation in the learning process. Simulation is suited to a constructivist approach as it is highly experiential, requiring mental and physical activity and affords the opportunity for reflection. Enacting a scenario provides the learner with the platform to learn through demonstrating the application of previous knowledge and skills in a novel situation.

Constructivism is very useful to simulation educators during debriefing. As learners try to make sense of the simulation activity and translate experience into learning, they draw from their own thoughts, motivations and prior experiences. A constructivist approach to debriefing promotes a facilitation of understanding rather than transmission of information. The educator provides the platform on which the learning takes place. Didactic learning is minimised and the learner's concerns take central focus. This core stance, drawn from learning theory, can be applied across different debriefing situations and is independent of a specific debriefing model (Box 7.1).

Social cognitive theory

Social cognitive theory (SCT) is primarily Albert Bandura's work and is congruent with constructivism. Bandura seeks to link the personal or cognitive aspect of learning with resulting behaviours and the environment, arguing that all three are necessarily interrelated. Most usefully, Bandura's theories consider 'human agency' (a person's capacity to determine how they respond within particular situation) to be central to learning (Bandura, 2001).

Two key concepts in SCT are 'self-efficacy' and 'self-regulation', both of which Bandura (2001) suggests are essential to learning. Self-efficacy is the belief that the learner can achieve the goal set before them; self-regulation is the means whereby a learner manages their cognitive and affective responses towards a learning orientation. Some of the key applications of these theories to SBE can be considered in scenario design. SCT suggests that offering learners opportunities which enhance their self-efficacy and allowing them to work at the right level of challenge enables learning. This is the opposite to the 'sink or swim' mentality. Additionally, simulation designs and associated debriefings can optimise opportunities for learners to regulate their own cognitive and emotional response to challenges. This type of capacity may assist learners to move towards using self-regulation as part of their professional practice (Box 7.2).

Situated learning theory

Situated learning theory privileges the value of the situation or context within which knowledge is learned. It suggests that all knowledge is contextual; not only is it grounded in a particular time and place, but the knowledge itself is actually co-produced by the moment of learning (Brown et al., 1989). Situated learning suggests we should think about how the practice environment is represented in SBE. This may be a call for more 'authenticity' within the scenario, so that the simulation scenario parallels the practice environment in the 'right ways'. It may also suggest that in some instances SBE may not be the right arena for learning areas of practice, or that in situ simulation may be optimal (Box 7.3).

Situated learning theory reinforces the need for educators and learners to highlight and manage the ways in which the 'real' practice environment will vary from the simulated learning environment. Yardley et al. (2013) refer to this as being 'mindful of the gap'.

Activity theory

Activity theory considers practices to be formed around a series of relationships between objects, instruments, subjects, divisions of labour, community and rules (Engestrom, 2000). These abstract concepts can be illustrated with a simple example. Consider a patient getting travel vaccines at a general practice. The object of this activity system is the patient's health and instruments include the vaccine, the syringe and the electronic health record. The subjects may be the general practitioner, the practice nurse and the patient. The labour is clearly divided, the patient tells the nurse about their proposed travel and previous history, the doctor checks the request and the nurse administers the vaccine. There are written rules which govern how the vaccine is administered and also unwritten rules such as handover information. Change of practice or learning can occur where there are serious contradictions within the activity system – in our example, the doctor may never provide advice and the practised division of labour may be in conflict with the actual rules. Contradictions may emerge in simulation scenarios and be highlighted in debriefings. Simulation facilitators and participants can promote learning through overtly reconciling those contradictions that have become problematic (Box 7.4). Battista (2017) offers an example of activity theory applied to simulation design.

For many health professionals, the acquisition and retention of both basic and high level technical skills is essential, not only in the 'craft specialties' such as surgery, but in other specialties and professions (radiography, midwifery, etc.). Learners need time to acquire proficiency in technical skills and it is no longer acceptable for learners to practise procedures on very sick, frail or vulnerable patients.

Acquiring proficiency and expertise in any technical skill requires the following:
• An underpinning knowledge and understanding of why the procedure is being done.
• A clear demonstration of how to carry out the procedure.
• Supervised, deliberate, purposeful, repetitive practise until the skill is mastered.
• Constructive feedback throughout.
• Sign off by an authorised person.

Simulation is widely used to help facilitate the learning required to attain the appropriate level of dexterity. This enables learners to acquire and retain vital technical skills (Ericsson, 2004) and helps to ensure that a learner's first human interaction in performing this skill is safe and effective (Aggarwal et al., 2010). Technical skill simulators range from clinical skills models and part task trainers (PTTs) (e.g. catheterisation, lumbar puncture) through to haptic feedback simulators.

Part task trainers

Part task trainers (PTTs) are commonly used in clinical skills laboratories, especially in the early stages of clinical learning. When planning training, each technical skill is either broken down into its component parts (e.g. elements of a surgical procedure) or is a discrete skill in its own right (e.g. cannulation). PTTs provide the essential components of the skill. They do not fully replicate the clinical encounter, but allow the learner to acquire the basic skills required to attempt performance in the clinical environment. Many innovative solutions have been developed in low resource settings, e.g. basic skills such as intramuscular injections can be practised on household objects such as sponges or pieces of fruit. Other PTTs include cannulation 'arms' for vascular access; a section of the spine for lumbar puncture; phantom heads for inserting an airway or dental work; body parts for ultrasound; and pelvic trainers for obstetrics, gynaecological procedures and catheterisation. PTTs are usually used in combination with real life clinical procedure equipment to help create a more realistic replication of a technical skill (Figure 13.1).

Animal training models and cadavers

Animal training models and human cadavers are used for dissection and for advanced procedural skills, e.g. prosthetic insertion. Increasingly, prosected specimens and virtual reality (VR) are used for anatomy teaching at undergraduate level, but cadavers still have a use in postgraduate training. Whilst both offer a high fidelity experience for certain technical skills, they are costly, require special facilities and licensing, and require ethical consideration.

Hybrid simulation

Hybrid simulation involves an actor working in combination with a PTT, e.g. a simulated patient has a plastic arm attached to them with a drape to allow a venous cannulation to be performed. The learner should have practised relevant skills in the skills laboratory before moving to this more expensive simulation. Hybrid simulation allows the learner to experience, practise and get feedback (from patient and trainer) on cannulation skills alongside communication skills with the patient simultaneously.

Virtual reality simulators

Advances in technology have demonstrated the potential for enhancing skills training. Many VR systems are available that allow more detailed measurement of learner performance (precision, accuracy, speed and error rates) and feedback than is possible in the real world. VR simulators are widely used, e.g. in minimally invasive surgery, where surgeons are guided by video images whilst using and manipulating instruments with limited degrees of freedom (Gallagher & Cates, 2004).

Haptic virtual reality simulators

Haptic feedback is where tactile feedback, in the form of vibrations, motions and a sense of a touch upon force application, is provided. This is very helpful in a range of situations, including where surgeons are using minimally invasive techniques and manipulating long wires or instruments. The 'operator has to adapt to significantly decreased tactile sensation and overcome … proprioceptive-visual conflict issues [and] combine to create substantial challenges' for those learning such skills (Gallagher & Cates, 2004).

Technical simulators at various levels of complexity are widely available. Many are coupled with educational prompts and graded exercises that increase in complexity to allow learners to master different skills. Individual account records of scores enable learners/trainers to monitor improvements. Multiple system-related simulators are now available. Cardiovascular procedures in the form of angiography, ultrasound and procedure rehearsal studios are used to create a patient-specific 3D virtual anatomical model based on a computed tomography (CT) scan, allowing the evaluation and practice of surgical treatment options (Figure 13.2a). Monitors visualise the procedure underpinned by computer software applications, which can be programmed to change the 'patient' responses to simulate a range of common or unusual situations. Respiratory, gastrointestinal, surgical, urological and orthopaedic simulators facilitate the following skills: bronchoscopy, endoscopy, laparoscopic procedures, transurethral resection of prostate and arthroscopy (Figure 13.2b–f). Simulated robotic surgery allows surgeons to master a range of procedures (Figure 13.2d) although sufficient simulation training must be undertaken before the surgeon operates the robotic surgical system 'for real' (Rajanbabu et al., 2014).

Combining simulators to create a simulated clinical scenario

Combining different simulators can support learners to utilise technical skills across a care pathway or situation, e.g. a hybrid simulation combining a haptic VR simulator and PTT allows a patient to have venepuncture before a bronchoscopy. The learner then moves to the bronchoscope console and an actor plays the part of a nurse, allowing the skills of multidisciplinary team communication to be mastered alongside the technical skill.

Summary

Technical skill simulators are widely used to help learners acquire basic and complex clinical skills, and learn new procedures. Through removing the real patient from the 'procedure', learners can concentrate on mastering technical skills, practise safely and as many times as they need to before they work with real patients and transfer the skills into clinical practice.

14 Manikins

Practice points

- Manikins have anatomical replicas of all or parts of the human body for the purposes of education
- The features and configuration of manikins are tailored to intended use and costs
- There is crossover between manikins that are designed to fulfil specific purposes and part task trainers

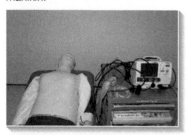

Figure 14.1 Basic resuscitation manikin.

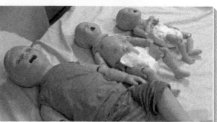

Figure 14.2 Range of paediatric manikins (child, newborn, premature).

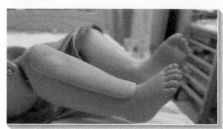

Figure 14.3 Intraosseous access in child mannikin.

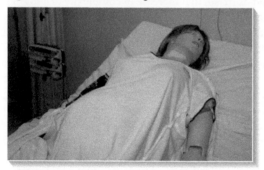

Figure 14.4 Obstetric emergencies manikin.

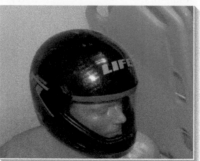

Figure 14.5 High fidelity trauma manikin.

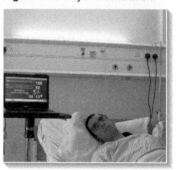

Figure 14.6 Hybrid simulation.

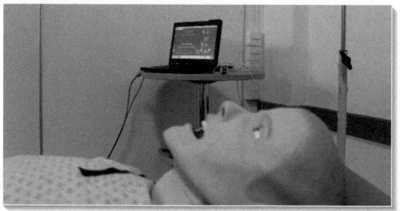

Figure 14.7 Manikin with wireless controller.

Box 14.1 Example features of high technology manikins.

Physiological replication	Pulses, strength responsive to blood pressure • Sweating, urinating • Pupil responses • Voice • Seizure • CO_2 exhalation • Heart, lung and bowel sounds
Programming, scenario and debriefing features	• Automated data collection for debriefing • Electrocardiogram generation and defibrillation/pacing responsive • Programmable scenarios • NFC (near field communication) enabled cannula • Able to perform invasive procedures

Box 14.2 Types of manikin.

Obstetric	• Anatomy of birthing canal, ability to simulate unique complications of pregnancy and birthing
Preterm/term infant	• Miniaturised manikin which replicates physiology of new born/premature
Child	• Common paediatric emergencies
Adult trauma	• Ruggedised and optimised for outdoor and trauma scenarios
Cardiopulmonary resuscitation	• Resuscitation trainer with a focus on basic and advanced life support (BLS/ALS)
Adult general	• Comprehensive feature set
Ultrasound trainer	• Ultrasoundable areas of anatomy, often to guide invasive procedures, with replaceable 'puncture blocks'

Healthcare Simulation at a Glance. First Edition. Kirsty Forrest and Judy McKimm. © 2019 John Wiley & Sons, Ltd.
Published 2019 by John Wiley & Sons, Ltd.

Static anatomical models have existed for centuries. In the mid-20th century, the first manikins with inbuilt physiological function began to appear. The well-known Resusci Annie (Laerdal Medical) was released in 1960, followed in the late 1960s by Sim One and HARVEY, the first to offer programmable physiological features such as pulses and respiration. Development of manikins has continued to advance in the intervening years, but equally important has been the rise in understanding and adoption of simulation as a learning method and how best to apply these technologies (Cooper & Taqueti, 2004).

Fidelity and technology

The existing technology in commercially available manikins has advanced greatly in recent years. At the most basic level, resuscitation trainers that allow for cardiopulmonary resuscitation (CPR) and airway manipulation are available. (Figure 14.1). These can often be augmented with electronic sensors that provide real time feedback on the quality of CPR. At the other end of the scale are wireless high technology models that are able to replicate a wide variety of physiological functions, and are programmable to follow predetermined scenarios or respond to learner actions in a defined way (Box 14.1).

Paediatric manikins carry a similar feature set to their adult counterparts, albeit with compromises related to their reduced size such as reduced battery performance or wireless control range (Figures 14.2 and 14.3). More specialist manikins are also available, such as those designed for obstetric or ultrasound training. (Figure 14.4). Their range of features is much narrower, in line with their intended use, although they are not part task trainers per se (Box 14.2).

Whilst manikins are frequently described as 'high fidelity', this is usually a measure of the technological sophistication (Figure 14.5). Fidelity should be applied in how they are used and the scenario environment. High technology manikins may be very useful in complex scenarios, and are capable of providing a wealth of data to feedback during debriefing, but their level of complexity may detract from the scenario in certain circumstances (Beaubien & Baker, 2004).

Hybrid simulation

There are several clinical scenarios that even the most advanced current manikins are unable to replicate with high fidelity. These include the nuance of a consultation with verbal and non-verbal communication cues and some neurological disorders. For these purposes, an actor or standardised patient is likely to offer a more realistic experience, but without the physiological changes. There is increasing interest in the use of hybrid simulation; blending features of simulation methods such as the use of an actor with a simulated monitor screen and manikin arm to optimise the fidelity (Figure 14.6) (Noeller et al., 2008).

Usage

Except for resuscitation training, the most common use of the manikin is during a simulation scenario. Entire scenarios can be pre-programmed into the software, or parameters can be altered on an ad hoc basis dependent on learner action. Even when pre-programmed, a faculty member is still required to operate the simulator to react to unexpected actions, and to act as the voice of the patient. In addition to baseline physiological parameters, setting up the manikin will often require physical adornment with clothing, medical equipment or moulage. A manikin in isolation is unlikely to provide the required degree of immersion and hence it is important to consider the environment in which it will be used. One major advantage of the current generation of self-contained wireless simulators is the ease with which they can be transported and used in situ (Figure 14.7).

The ability to connect to a manikin wirelessly enables more creative scenario design, where the scenario can move through clinical areas, or occur in outdoor or difficult to access areas. Battery life is typically 3–4 hours, and wireless range is typically 10 m or greater. Pre-programmed scenarios are available to purchase.

Debriefing with manikins

The most advanced manikins are able to collect a wide range of timed metrics during the scenario to assist with debriefing. Examples include the sequence of physical examination correlated with observations, name, dose and rate of drug given, and duration and quality of chest compressions, with time and energy of defibrillation. Software tools are available to integrate manikin outputs and video-assisted debriefing set-ups.

Summary

The most important consideration when selecting a manikin is the intended usage. Those looking to develop advanced simulations for a wide variety of learners may be best served with a general purpose, high technology model. Those with simpler needs, or a limited budget, may be able to design effective scenarios using a lower technology model. The environment in which a manikin is to be used, the need for portability and in situ use and the level of facilitator expertise should all be considered. The availability of pre-programmed scenarios for the model may be of value to some. Creative use of moulage and adjuncts, and using a hybrid approach is likely to result in improved learning.

15 Audio and video recording

Figure 15.1 Video to assist in the debriefing process.

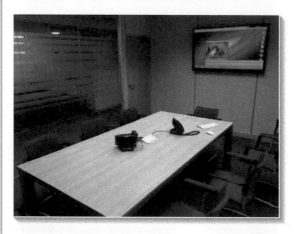

Figure 15.2 Streaming to another room to engage a larger group.

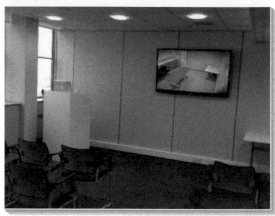

Figure 15.3 Complex technology.

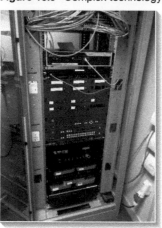

Figure 15.4 Cameras.

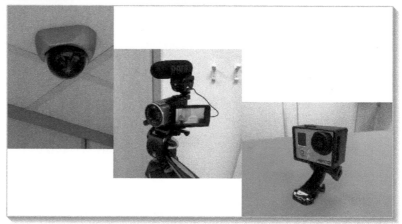

Figure 15.5 Portable equipment.

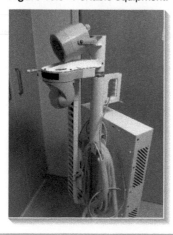

Figure 15.6 WiFi network.

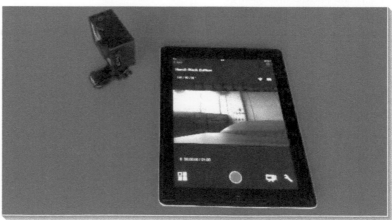

Healthcare Simulation at a Glance. First Edition. Kirsty Forrest and Judy McKimm. © 2019 John Wiley & Sons, Ltd.
Published 2019 by John Wiley & Sons, Ltd.

Audio-visual (AV) streaming and recording is facilitated for a number of reasons in simulation-based learning events. This includes using video to assist in the debriefing process (Figure 15.1), streaming to another room to engage a larger group (Figure 15.2), for research, and to allow summative assessments to be verified. The use of AV recording raises issues around confidentiality and concerns around the security of stored media. Explicit consent needs to be gained from participants, explaining who will be permitted to view the resources and how these will be stored.

There is currently a lack of evidence to suggest that video-assisted debriefing outcomes are significantly improved over non-video-assisted ones (Cheng et al., 2014) but it continues to be widely used in simulation sessions. The use of AV systems adds another layer of complexity for simulation faculty. A wide range of levels of technology (and associated costs) can be used, with some of these systems being very complex (Figure 15.3). Consultation, advice and support from organisational IT departments will be required in order to integrate systems with one another and ensure maintenance and replacement.

Video cameras and audio capture

There is a range of available cameras that include web cams, small point of view cameras, fixed ceiling mounted cameras and freestanding cameras (Figure 15.4). As well as the range of physical camera types there are a number of camera recording resolutions. When deciding the resolution required, it is important to consider the cost, what is being viewed and the device on which the video will be viewed. If we are watching individual interactions, then lower resolution cameras are often sufficient; however if we are watching an intricate clinical procedure, then higher resolution may be required. Often microphones are incorporated into the camera but additional external microphones may be provided, either worn by learners or, more often, ceiling mounted in suitable locations (e.g. over the patient's trolley). Audio pick-ups may also be used on telephones allowing both sides of calls to be heard.

AV transmission

The transmission of the AV signal depends on the camera type and outputs. As well as recording audio from the simulation, there is often a requirement for speech to be transmitted from the control room – although not all manikins have this option. A video feed from the patient monitor may also be transmitted.

For simple systems, the camera connects directly to the computer by a suitable cable. Another common option is to send the AV signal over an existing local area network (LAN). Portable equipment (Figure 15.5) can be purchased that connects to LANs and allows remote control of cameras, the option of transmitting several video channels and two-way audio. Sometimes a more flexible solution, especially for mobile simulation, is to stream over a wifi network (Figure 15.6).

AV storage

If the AV signal needs to be recorded, then the storage requirements depend on the method of transmission and the needs of the users. Files can be stored in an array of formats with a variety of associated file sizes. It is important to ensure that the format is the correct type for all the programs that may use it. A camera connected directly to a computer can record to its hard drive. Some cameras can record onto memory cards, however the physical removal of these cards can hinder the rapid turnaround sometimes required. When cameras are connected to a LAN, a variety of storage solutions including dedicated local servers and external servers accessed via the internet will be required, including being able to access these servers from a variety of computers. Most organisations will have policies about files being stored external to firewalls and this will often be a heightened issue where the storage is out of the country (e.g. cloud-based solutions).

Where multiple AV signals (several cameras, monitors and audio feeds) are used, the audio levels will need to be balanced and a method to view several video feeds on the same screen will have to be provided. This is often done with equipment that provides an image in picture view. It is often this feed that is recorded and streamed as required.

AV playback

The final stage is the playback of the material. It is important to consider how the video will be utilised in the debriefing. Is the entire video clip to be shown? There may be times, especially with shorter simulations, where this is useful as it give participants the opportunity to observe what was happening around them. However, often this is not the most productive use of valuable time. Another possibility is to note the time of particular events and fast forward to that point – however this often ends up with more time spent fast forwarding and rewinding the video than debriefing. A final solution is to tag or electronically mark the video, either as it is recorded or retrospectively, so when the participant asks, 'Did I manage the airway appropriately?', the facilitator can instantly play the appropriate part of the video. Some systems are flexible enough for the tagging to include a performance rating allowing specific areas of development or areas of best performance to be demonstrated. Tagging allows the AV use to become responsive to the debriefing questions rather than steering the debrief.

16 Learning technologies and simulation

Practice points

- Evolving technology has led to many developments in simulation education
- Immersive technologies, wearable technologies and serious games have huge applicability to healthcare simulation
- Due to fast-changing technology, learning analytics is a rapidly expanding area of research

Figure 16.1 Virtual patient.

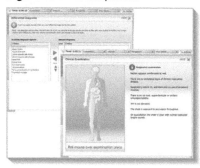

Figure 16.2 Dome and CAVE.

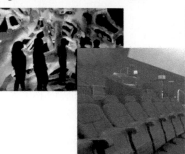

Figure 16.3 Holographic simulation using Microsoft Hololense.

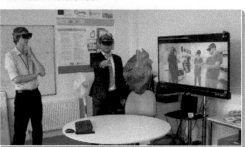

Figure 16.4 Serious game for ebola infection prevention and control.

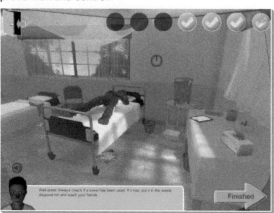

Figure 16.5 Gamification.

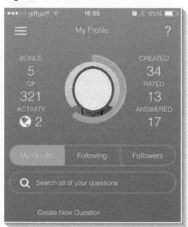

Figure 16.6 Wearables.

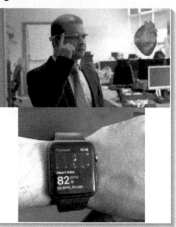

Figure 16.7 Analytics.

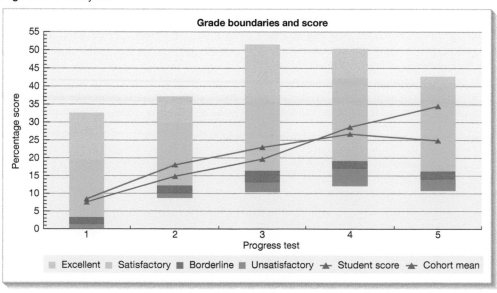

Healthcare Simulation at a Glance. First Edition. Kirsty Forrest and Judy McKimm. © 2019 John Wiley & Sons, Ltd.
Published 2019 by John Wiley & Sons, Ltd.

The wider educational landscape has witnessed a paradigm shift in the last few decades from a predominantly transmissive pedagogy to a more transformative pedagogy. An important contributing factor for this shift is the evolving technological landscape and its affordability. Simulation-based education (SBE) is no different and some of the key learning technologies used for simulation are outlined here.

Virtual patients

Virtual patients (VPs) enable learners to experience simulated patient conditions, which they may not otherwise encounter during their studies (Figure 16.1). Learners usually interact with actual patient data, then piece together a full diagnosis and detailed treatment plan. VPs allow for immersion and realism to a varying degree of fidelity by incorporating audio and video content, still imagery and interactive objects. VPs allow students to learn from their mistakes by making meaning from experience, and allowing them to actively experiment without disadvantaging or harming a real patient. VPs can be used across several competency domains but are primarily used for clinical reasoning, procedural skills and patient communication. Interactive and linear VPs do not necessarily require dedicated software. For example, you could use Moodle lessons or PowerPoint with TurningPoint clickers to 'go through' the patients and discuss the case, diagnoses and treatment options. Developing non-linear VPs (i.e. with options and algorithms) is more complicated and Openlabyrinth.ca is a good place to start exploring this. However, it can become time consuming to create a non-linear comprehensive VP.

Immersive technologies

By definition, immersion involves a user experiencing multiple features of a simulated environment as if it is real. To achieve this, various devices and approaches use multimodal techniques creating the necessary sensory stimuli. This section covers the two main types of immersive environments.

Domes and CAVEs

The cinematic environment of planetarium full domes and CAVEs (cave automatic virtual environments) (Figure 16.2) lends itself to projecting dramatic material in a new and engaging way, totally absorbing the participant in the 'show'. This unique opportunity can be used to great effect, providing health improvement messages and to simulate physiological developments and reactions which are meaningful to the audience. Additionally, portable domes allow immersive and distributed simulation to be carried out in in remote locations.

Head-mounted displays and holograms

A 3D inertial sensor (IS) uses a customised algorithm developed by Oculus VR to track and monitor head movement so the content displayed can reflect an immersive virtual reality environment. Technologies like Oculus Rift allow a learner to be fully immersed in a clinical scenario and interact with it. Similarly, the upcoming Microsoft Hololense enables augmented reality simulations (Figure 16.3).

Serious games

Learning through visual and competitive systems using the latest technology (in the form of digital games) is fast becoming a popular teaching method for complex subjects and methods that need to be remembered. Interactive health-related games (Figure 16.4) are increasingly being used to foster learning as they effectively activate engagement using intrinsic (entertainment) and extrinsic motivators and help simulate a sense of achievement (badges, game levels, etc.) while attaining the learning objectives. Within health, serious games are predominantly used for:

- medical error avoidance
- rehabilitation processes
- repetitive tasks.

In addition to dedicated health-based games, the concept of *gamification* is being increasingly used within simulation enhanced education. Gamification applies the mechanics of gaming to non-game activity (Figure 16.5) to change people's behaviour.

Wearable technologies

Technologies such as smart watches, helmets, glasses and garments are pushing the boundaries further, providing the ability to factor in the learner's action and motion (Figure 16.6). The key principle is to gather real time data about and around the user in an unobtrusive manner, subsequently analysing and presenting it back to the user to act upon. For example, smart glasses have been used for facilitating live remote observation during surgical procedures and remote consultations. Smart watches with sensors to monitor health data provide further opportunities to converge various data points during simulation enhanced sessions.

Learning analytics

As a result of fast-changing technological standards, the semantic web, data mining and big data, the possibility of capturing learning events within simulated settings, store and analyse them in conjunction with data from other sources is now plausible. Learning analytics (LA) is a rapidly evolving body of research with the aim of providing a more personalised learning experience. In their systematic review, Papamitsiou and Economides (2014) highlight the potential of improving learner behaviours, and reflective practice, with resulting performance prediction and appropriate use of resources. Typically, processed data are presented to the learner using visualisation dashboards, as shown in Figure 16.7. Some key evolving considerations are around the ethical use of learner data, data storage and storing the data within relevant institutions, e.g. the learner's present or future employers.

17 Distributed simulation

Practice points

- Distributed simulation (DS) is an affordable, portable, self-contained immersive form of simulation
- DS comprises the simulation environment, clinical props and the audio-visual control room
- Drawing on psychological concepts, DS has strong validity and can easily incorporate a variety of clinical challenges
- Sequential simulation (SqS Simulation™) uses DS to simulate a number of care pathways and settings

Figure 17.1 DS inflatable structure and lamp.

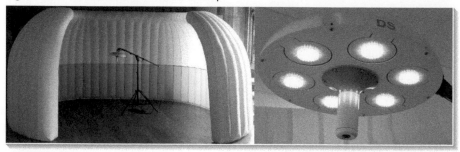

Figure 17.2 DS pull-up backdrops.

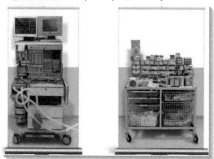

Figure 17.3 Inflatable structure with lamp and backdrops.

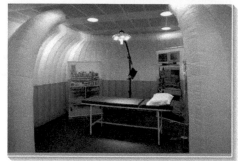

Figure 17.4 DS components packed.

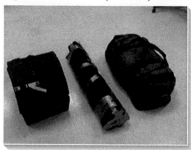

Figure 17.5 DS software interface.

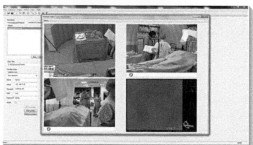

Figure 17.6 A terminally ill patient care pathway, SqS simulation™.

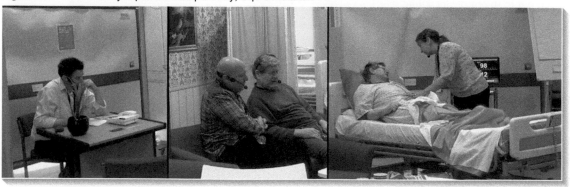

Healthcare Simulation at a Glance. First Edition. Kirsty Forrest and Judy McKimm. © 2019 John Wiley & Sons, Ltd.
Published 2019 by John Wiley & Sons, Ltd.

Distributed simulation (DS) refers to affordable, portable and accessible, self-contained immersive simulation (Kneebone et al., 2010). DS seeks to optimise the level of fidelity by selecting and recreating only the most salient features of a clinical setting that provide the key cues necessary for engaging participants and achieving the desired educational outcomes. The design concept of DS draws on theories of attention in cognitive psychology and is based on the 'circles of focus' model (Kneebone, 2010), which describes the concentric nature of participants' selective perception, awareness and attention to the different elements that make up a clinical setting within a simulation.

DS components

A DS system comprises three main components: the simulation environment, the clinical props and the audio-visual (AV) control room. This is similar in function to a traditional static simulation facility, but with the advantages of portability, flexibility and accessibility; and all at an affordable cost.

The DS simulation environment consists of a self-contained, enclosable space provided by retractable screens or inflatable structures that create a boundary in clinical training that establishes the context for education and professional practice (Figure 17.1). Inside the inflatable structure, vital items of clinical equipment such as trolleys, instrument cupboards, anaesthetic machines, patient beds, etc. are represented through high-resolution pull-up backdrops, custom-built props or off the shelf products (Figure 17.2). For example, a lightweight, custom-designed, portable operating lamp mounted on a standard tripod represents a crucial component of an operating theatre DS simulation environment (Figures 17.1 and 17.3). Although considerably smaller and lighter than a standard operating lamp, the protable lamp's circular shape, adjustable position and multiple bright lights adequately recreate a real operating lamp in both appearance and function. A video camera and microphone in the central handle record interactions in the operative field. Additional items of equipment (e.g. instrument trays, crash trolley) may be brought inside the DS simulation environment as necessary.

Due to the portable nature of the DS simulation environment, it can be easily set up by two people in under an hour, and packed up in less than 30 minutes. All key components can be transported in a car or van, depending on the number of scenarios to be recreated. The operating theatre example in Figure 17.3 can be fitted into the boot of a small car (Figure 17.4).

DS can include a portable AV control room from which the simulation can be observed and managed without disruption. This consists of wireless cameras, a laptop computer, lightweight speakers and bespoke recording and playback software capable of real time recording. The wireless cameras complement the video camera integrated in the DS lamp, but could also be integrated into other parts of a DS recreation. Within the DS lamp, the cameras can be positioned within the DS enclosure to offer a wide range of different views to satisfy individual learning and teaching needs, with recording of team interaction and team performance. Audio cues are recreated in the DS simulation environment through small loudspeakers hidden within the contextual structure. Playback of a variety of clinical sounds (e.g. heart monitor, ventilator, clinical background noise) may be controlled from the laptop computer in the portable AV control room.

Figure 17.5 shows a snapshot of the DS software interface.

The evidence

DS has been shown to have strong face, content and construct validity, offering a valid, low cost, accessible environment for training and assessing surgeons (Kassab et al., 2011; Brewin et al., 2012). A separate study showed that it is perceived as a better training tool for clinical education than traditional bench-top models, suggesting that it should be integrated after bench-top training and before practising in a real operating theatre (Kassab et al., 2012). Tun et al. (2012) demonstrated that, by systematically designing simulations using the principles of DS, clinical challenge can be effectively incorporated into simulations.

Sequential simulation

Building on DS, the concept of *sequential simulation* (SqS Simulation™) frames clinical care as a *sequence* of interconnected events rather than a single episode (Weldon et al., 2015a, 2015b). By selecting representative components of a clinical trajectory and linking them together, SqS Simulation™ invites participants to identify which components of a care pathway are critical for the objectives at hand. Designing scenarios based on established care pathways, known sequences of care, and patient and clinician's experiences, DS is drawn on to recreate the identified clinical settings through the identification of contexts (clinical backdrops), props, actors (for the patient roles) and real clinicians. SqS Simulation™ can be used for training purposes but also allows care pathways to be viewed, challenged and remodelled as a collaborative endeavour (Figure 17.6).

SqS Simulation™ is flexible and can be undertaken in most settings. The emphasis is therefore on the ability of the scenarios to achieve the desired objectives and not on the facilities available (e.g. simulation suites), which can often be expensive, inaccessible or not designed to accommodate simulations that require more than one clinical setting at a time. SqS Simulation™ has the potential to simulate an infinite number of scenarios and care pathways. Its application is wide and healthcare practitioners, managers, funders and patients are seeing the benefit of such an approach for a range of activities from pre-intervention evaluations and clinical training, to public and patient involvement and quality improvement projects (Huddy et al., 2016; Kneebone et al., 2016; Powell, et al., 2016; Weldon et al., 2016; Tribe, 2018; Weil et al., 2018).

18 Engagement and simulation science

Figure 18.1 Engagement and simulation science.

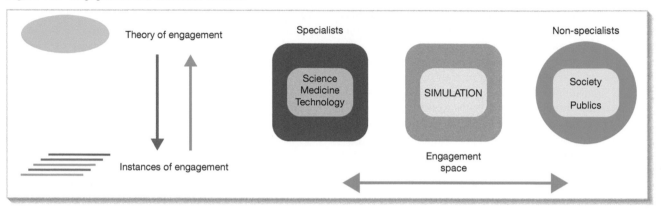

Figure 18.2 Engagement space.

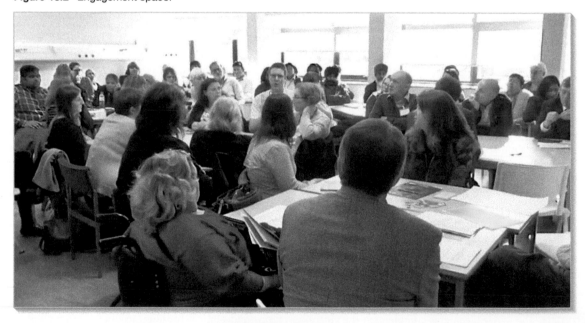

Figure 18.3 A diabetic patient care pathway SqS Simulation™.

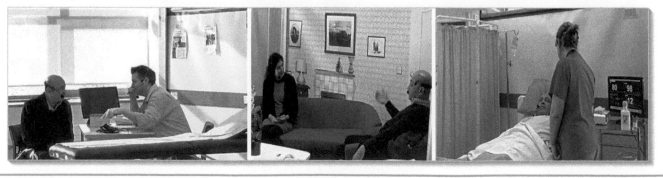

Healthcare Simulation at a Glance. First Edition. Kirsty Forrest and Judy McKimm. © 2019 John Wiley & Sons, Ltd.
Published 2019 by John Wiley & Sons, Ltd.

Engagement and simulation science (ESS) is a rapidly evolving field which is opening new horizons for simulation practice and research.

Concept of engagement

Most healthcare simulation is framed as a means of training clinical professionals, whether as students or later in their careers. Emphasis is on learning how to carry out procedures or operations. Patients are *represented* (by simulators, manikins, models or professional actors), but seldom take part themselves. Indeed, ensuring safety by excluding real patients is key to simulator design.

Discussions around healthcare are difficult within the context of the care itself. There, the focus is rightly on individual patients and their needs rather than on reshaping pathways. Moreover, power differentials between professionals and patients can make candid discussion difficult. But healthcare is not exclusive to professionals. It concerns us all (as members of society) as well as affecting us at a personal level (when we or those we care about become ill). Yet when we do become patients or carers, our voices are often drowned out by those of so-called experts.

Improvements in healthcare cannot be brought about by healthcare professionals alone. The challenges are joint and solutions can only be found through collaboration. Yet the experiences of patients, carers, clinicians, managers and policy makers are very different, and healthcare innovations often fail because they do not involve all stakeholders. Interaction is the cornerstone of healthcare (Figure 18.1).

Engagement space

We call this interaction 'engagement'. This is different from the more specific term 'public or patient engagement', with its resonances of knowledgeable experts dispensing information about completed work in a largely one-way transmission. Instead of dividing people into 'experts' (such as clinicians) or 'non-experts' (such as patients or those who care for them), we propose that all participants possess expertise. Though the expertise of performing surgery, for example, is very different from the expertise of undergoing it, every viewpoint is valid and all are important.

Engagement in this sense involves sharing expertise – a respectful exchange of perspectives aimed at bringing about *reciprocal illumination* (Kneebone, 2015). Here we explore how simulation can mediate between different worlds of experience, creating 'working models' of clinical care that can be refined collaboratively.

We propose that simulation be seen not only in terms of simulators and kit, but as the means of connection with an *engagement space* (Figure 18.2). As well as ensuring safety from physical harm, this can allow clinicians to see themselves as their patients see them and to make the healthcare system more transparent. To succeed, however, simulation must ring true for all participants.

Most simulation takes place in simulation centres, where access is tightly restricted to authorised staff. It can be almost as difficult to enter a simulated operating theatre or intensive care unit as a real one. This chapter proposes an alternative view, where simulation becomes a means of inviting non-professionals in rather than keeping them out.

Engagement through simulation

The concepts of distributed simulation (DS) and sequential simulation (SqS Simulation™) open new possibilities (Kneebone, 2010; Kneebone et al., 2010; Kassab et al., 2011; Weldon et al., 2015a; see also Chapter 17). For example, DS allows realistic simulation to be provided in any suitable area (including public spaces), while SqS Simulation™ recreates pathways of care and invites participants to 'sketch out' possible changes through enactment. In more than a hundred engagement events over the past decade we have explored how simulation can connect professionals and the public around clinical practice and biomedical science. These range from large-scale performances at major museums and science fairs to small groups in community settings.

Examples include elective and emergency coronary intervention; adolescent asthma; frail elderly patients with complex medical and social challenges; emergency surgery for abdominal trauma; the introduction of cutting-edge bioscience into clinical medicine; and a range of technology-based approaches based on sophisticated haptics. In each case simulation-based scenarios have been developed in conjunction with patients and the public.

An example of care pathway modelling

A group of 65 people (including patients, carers, clinicians and care managers) come together to develop better ways of designing care within the UK NHS. An SqS Simulation™ scenario, developed from the real-life experiences of patients and clinicians, shows a middle-aged man with poorly controlled diabetes and social issues using low-cost props to recreate the patient's home, their family doctor's consulting room and a hospital ward. The simulation shows the patient and his wife seeing his GP, a specialist nurse and other healthcare professionals in a system where communication is dysfunctional (Figure 18.3) (Weldon et al., 2016).

The audience then splits into groups and they come up with suggestions for improving this enacted pathway. A week later and an increase in participants (to 93), these suggestions have been incorporated into a second SqS Simulation™ where a multidisciplinary gathering of 10 professionals assembles in the patient's home to discuss how best to integrate his care. At once the audience – who themselves came up with this proposal – recognise serious flaws. The patient is overwhelmed by all the experts in one sitting, his wife feels alienated, and the practical difficulties of assembling so many professionals at one time would be formidable; the list goes on. Further group discussion leads to new ideas and the process of reciprocal illumination continues. It was only by enactment through simulation that these issues became visible and could be addressed.

Engagement and simulation science

ESS is a young and vibrant field. While much current activity and literature around simulation is directed at professionals and insiders, ESS frames the public and patients as partners in co-production. The next stage is to map what engagement through simulation can offer, drawing on the rigorous methodologies of natural and social science. These are exciting times.

19 In situ and mobile simulation

Practice points

- Advantages of mobile simulation include increased authenticity, enabling practise with existing teams and infrastructure, and opportunities for innovation
- In situ simulation (ISS) involves blending simulated and real healthcare environments
- Many challenges exist, including the safety of real patients and enabling the involvement of a wide range of staff

Figure 19.1 Mobile simulation: control room set up in a hospital ward.

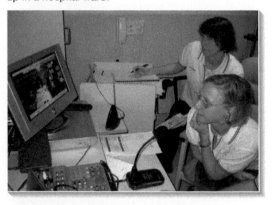

Figure 19.2 ISS in action.

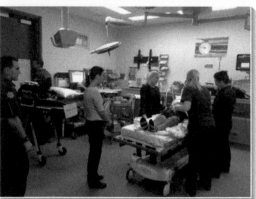

Box 19.1 Practical safety strategies for ISS.

- Pre-warning involved departments of the hospital and patients in adjoining cubicles
- Liaison with triage/floor team leaders about other patients and workload in the emergency department
- Signposting patient areas and beds being used as 'Simulation'
- Avoid using 'fake' or non-functioning equipment or drugs in clinical areas – they may be left behind and used on real patients
- Labelling documentation 'Simulation only'
- Providing simulated patients with advice about recognising safety risks, e.g. practitioner actually performing procedure
- Use of scenario confederates to recognise and prevent same risk
- Maintain patient confidentiality by avoiding camera angles in which real patients are captured
- Maintain high level of occupational health and safety (OHS) risk assessment – cables, electrical and pneumatic simulation equipment

Box 19.2 Case study: in situ stroke simulation.

The emergency department (ED) and neurology team in an large hospital decide to improve their performance in acute stroke care. As this involves complex interactions between teams, equipment and hospital processes, they decide to run a program of in situ simulation (ISS). The ISS involves a trained actor arriving by ambulance, paging systems being utilised to notify the stroke team, initial assessment being undertaken in ED, using usual equipment and staff, followed by rapid transfer to the computed tomography (CT) department and initiation of thrombolytic medication if indicated.

Note the involvement of paramedics, ED staff, wards persons, medical imaging staff, and the stroke team; and the use of monitoring equipment, transfer packs, and other equipment typically used for this patient.

Figure 19.3 ISS in action.

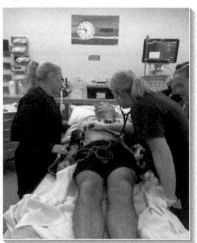

Figure 19.4 ISS in action.

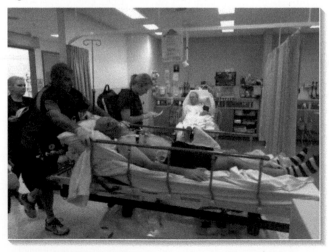

Healthcare Simulation at a Glance. First Edition. Kirsty Forrest and Judy McKimm. © 2019 John Wiley & Sons, Ltd.
Published 2019 by John Wiley & Sons, Ltd.

Mobile simulation

This is a broad term describing simulation-based education (SBE) delivery in a venue away from a simulation centre. This usually involves the transport of manikins and audio-visual equipment to a location where a temporary simulation environment is set up. In some cases this can include a mobile 'bus' in which the simulation area is permanently set up but transportable. Other techniques involve freighting equipment and setting up either in situ in a clinical area or in a non-clinical room.

This provides obvious advantages in accessibility of simulation training for healthcare teams to train together, and frequently allows them to use their own equipment and systems. Debriefing discussions can more effectively be targeted at the team and systems level, rather than the individual practitioner who attends a training course at a simulation centre.

However, the logistical challenges can be significant. Manikins are heavy and technologically fragile, and connecting cables suffer wear and tear with repeated connection and disconnection. Wifi-based connections may be problematic in unfamiliar clinical environments.

Audio-visual systems need to be flexible, and delivery teams need to include staff sufficiently skilled in their use. The team needs strategies to accommodate technical failures, including redundancy and alternative educational strategies.

Set-ups in non-clinical locations are especially challenging as the clinical equipment and environment need to be recreated, which is a high intensity exercise for a temporary venue. The inflatable 'operating theatre' illustrates one way to approach this challenge (Kneebone et al., 2010).

In situ simulation

In situ simulation (ISS) is a specific example of mobile simulation. It involves blending simulated and real healthcare working environments, e.g. by using a manikin or simulated patient scenario within a working emergency department, ward or operating theatre. This involves using all the standard equipment, medications, staff and care processes that would usually be applied to a 'real' patient in that area (Figure 19.1). This approach aims to improve transfer of training because of the increased physical resemblance and task fidelity of the simulation. However, the target for ISS is not just the individual healthcare provider's knowledge and skills. ISS ideally 'involves simulation that accounts for and is fully integrated with clinical operations, people, information technology and systems (Guise & Mladenovic, 2013). Posner et al. (2017) discuss the lexicon around SBE and describe not putting a value

judgement on the type of simulation but rather to decide on which delivery best fits the goals, needs and strengths of that modality.

Practical considerations

Delivery of ISS is challenging. The safety of other 'real' patients can be compromised by a focus on a simulation in the next room, or use of equipment, care processes or resources needed for real patients. Hospital services such as the blood bank or medical imaging may be 'activated' inadvertently without knowledge that the ISS is a simulation exercise. Damage or harm may occur to manikins because of intense 'immersion' of participants. Appropriate debriefing venues can be hard to identify as well. Issues related to safety and strategies used to overcome them are listed in Box 19.1 See Figures 19.2–19.4 for examples of ISS where the simulated patients are difficult to tell apart from the real patients when in the workplace.

Rosen et al. (2012) offer a multilevel framework for the needs addressed by ISS – individual, team, unit level and organisational outcomes. At the level of organisational outcomes, ISS can provide an opportunity for 'innovation and exploration to discover potential problems in the healthcare delivery system and test new methods of work'. For example, a multicentre intervention in obstetrics using ISS identified a systems issue in each hospital, including those related to communication, medication, environment, devices/equipment, staffing/roles and protocols. More significantly, institutions reported being able to identify and implement potential solutions once they were aware of the systems issues. See Box 19.2 for a single institution example.

Communication between healthcare teams is a crucial element of system performance and 'intergroup conflict' and healthcare tribalism is a specific challenge (Hewett et al., 2009). ISS can provide a venue to develop inter-team coordination skills and processes and to open discussion about fundamental conflicts between teams in an authentic way.

A literature review of current ISS practice (Rosen et al., 2012) described the method as relatively underdeveloped and called for more use of formal and rigorous needs analysis methods, specific training for ISS providers, greater explicit focus on the levels of performance addressed (e.g. individual, team and unit work system levels), more rigorous performance measurement practices, and improved evaluation practices.

A specific recommendation for practice was that:

> 'facilitation of in situ simulation session require different resources, planning, and data capture methods that traditional simulation settings; therefore, faculty development specific to in situ simulation may be required.' (Rosen et al., 2012)

20 Human factors

Figure 20.1 Example of a simulation.

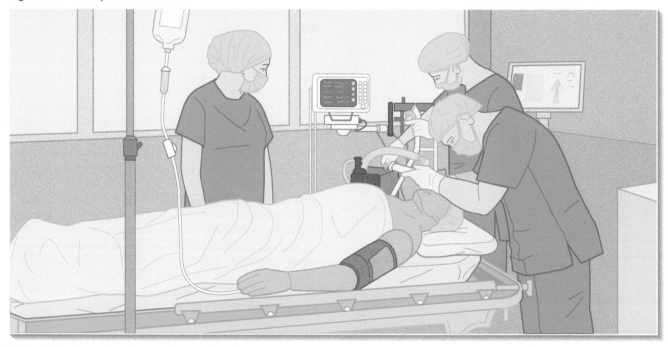

Table 20.1 Examples of human factors simulation scenarios.

Communication	Structured challenging communication scenarios including a mixture of verbal, telephone and written handovers
Fatigue and stress management	Multiple distraction scenario with several competing 'urgent' tasks to complete in a short time schedule
Distraction	Performance of a skilled procedural task with multiple interruptions ongoing
Decision making	Scenario where multiple courses of action are possible, with a 'think out loud' model employed to determine decision rationale
Authority gradient	In situ simulation using a team where issues with authority have been identified such as the presence of a domineering authority figure
Leadership	Scenario requiring the demonstration of effective leadership in order for successful completion such as coordinating an unfamiliar team to perform several tasks simultaneously, requiring the leader to step back and coordinate
Situational awareness	Scenario with rapidly changing environment which requires capture and interpretation of external information. Awareness of situation can be captured by pausing scenario at points to evaluate whether key markers have been recognised and acted upon

Healthcare Simulation at a Glance. First Edition. Kirsty Forrest and Judy McKimm. © 2019 John Wiley & Sons, Ltd.
Published 2019 by John Wiley & Sons, Ltd.

Human factors describes the study of the interface between humans and systems. The 'system' in a healthcare context could describe an individual piece of equipment or technology, an entire department, a hospital or a regional or national health system. Human factors are involved in all aspects of healthcare, and there is close interaction between the knowledge and technical skills required to deliver patient care and the way that they are carried out. The term ergonomics is used synonymously with human factors.

Human factors and errors

As humans, we have huge impact on healthcare through the importance of the decisions we make, our awareness of situations and the way we communicate within teams. Healthcare is an increasingly complex enterprise and a considerable number of patients will experience harm as a result of errors in their care. The importance of human factors in medical errors was recognised over 20 years ago. For example, in 1999 it was estimated that up to 98 000 people die in the United States per year as a result of error, costing up to $29 billion per year (CQHCA, 1999).

Many medical errors are not a failure of technical skill, competence or knowledge but are a combination of both technical and non-technical skills. We can use the information gained from errors that have occurred to identify points of weakness in systems and training needs for staff. Simulation has an important role to play in testing the interplay of human factors and systems through recreating adverse events that have happened in a safe manner (Figure 20.1). A number of reports have advocated the increasing use of simulation training in technical and non-technical skills and have emphasised the importance of human factors to reduce healthcare error and improve patient safety (Donaldson, 2008; World Alliance for Patient Safety, 2008).

Areas for improvement

The approach to human factors should not focus solely on one aspect of improvement, but rather should incorporate both staff training and system improvements simultaneously. Simulation can be used to good effect in this context. An example of this is in the design and building phases of a new hospital department. Virtual modelling could be used to simulate patient flow and emergency response requirements at design, and real-time in situ simulation could be used to train staff and identify unforeseen points of weakness or potential error sources prior to the opening.

A number of different concepts in human factors have been described, for example the World Health Organisation (WHO) identify the following topic areas: organisational culture, managerial leadership, communication, teamwork, team leadership, situational awareness, decision making, stress, fatigue and work environment (Flin et al., 2009). Other areas include distraction, decision making and the authority gradient. However, whilst these may be useful constructs in description and in the design of educational objectives for courses, in reality there is a great deal of overlap between them (Table 20.1).

Designing simulation with a human factors' focus

Although many simulation scenarios will involve an element of human factor observation, in order to gain maximum benefit, learning objectives and scenario design should be planned with specific learning needs in mind. As with any educational programme, a needs assessment is the first stage of development. Specific learning needs may be identified by clinical incidents, self-identified learning needs or observed performance.

The choice of simulation modality is important to consider when designing simulation scenarios for human factors' training. One method which is commonly used is in situ simulation, allowing learners to practise within their usual working environments using the equipment they are familiar with and in their usual teams. This can be particularly useful to recreate actual incidents and identify weak spots such as monitoring equipment being out of view or where protocol compliance is not possible.

More abstract methods can also be used to demonstrate human factors' principles when delivering simulation. Transferable skills such as dealing with distraction or accurate communication during crisis situations can be simulated through relatively straightforward scenarios, and debriefed with a focus on strategies for improving performance in these areas in similar situations. As with all simulation training, a focus on learner immersion and allowing them to reflect on normal patterns of behaviour in each scenario is important; false representation by the learner will result in ineffective attempts to change practice.

Video recording of simulation and targeted playback during debriefing may allow the learner to identify areas of unintentional practice. An example of this may be in evaluating verbal communication during a handover. The learner may intend to communicate in a clear, concise fashion and fail to recognise deficiencies until they are able to witness their own performance in the context of a facilitated debriefing.

Debriefing should be undertaken by experienced educators who have expertise in both the clinical aspects of the area of focus and also in identifying and debriefing human factors. Care should be taken to avoid excessive discussion of the technical aspects and losing focus of the human factors' learning outcomes.

Implementation

Programmes such as TeamSTEPPS® (AHRQ, 2015) are available to help educators who have identified specific human factors' learning needs. Existing simulation scenarios and programmes can also be adapted to incorporate specific human factors' learning objectives. Learners should be encouraged to reflect upon their experience and implement changes to practice, whereas organisations should be encouraged to implement system changes to reduce the risk of latent error.

21 Non-technical skills

Figure 21.1 Safe task performance can only be achieved through a combination of non-technical and technical skills.

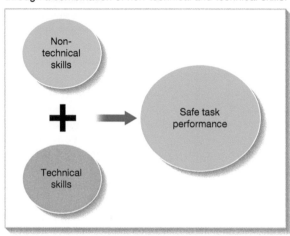

Figure 21.2 Non-technical skills training is important in improving safety in high risk environments such as aviation, nuclear power, the oil industry, the military and medicine.

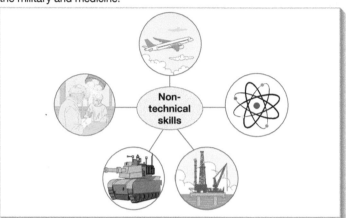

Figure 21.3 Non-technical skills include both cognitive and interpersonal domains.

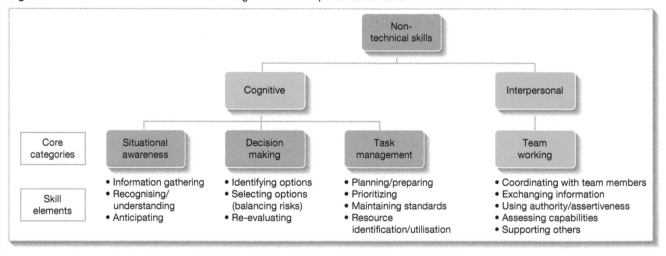

Figure 21.4 Situational awareness involves three stages: perception, comprehension and projection of future status.

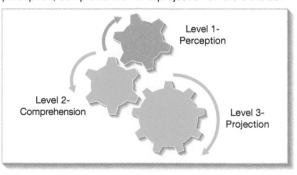

Healthcare Simulation at a Glance. First Edition. Kirsty Forrest and Judy McKimm. © 2019 John Wiley & Sons, Ltd.
Published 2019 by John Wiley & Sons, Ltd.

Non-technical skills comprise the cognitive and interpersonal domains that complement technical proficiency in enabling individuals to perform tasks safely and efficiently (Figure 21.1).

Historical perspective

'Human factors' refer to the ways in which individuals interact with the elements of a system in which they operate, including colleagues ('liveware'), guidelines and protocols ('software'), machines and computers ('hardware') and the working environment itself. In the 1970s, research into flight safety identified that the majority of accidents were due to human factors rather than technical inadequacies. In response to these findings the aviation industry introduced non-technical skills training for pilots, cabin crew and members of the air traffic control team as part of crew resource management (CRM). These CRM courses have resulted in a reduction in adverse outcomes and improved flight crew performance. Extrapolating from the aviation blueprint, CRM programmes have been successfully integrated into the training schemes for other high reliability work settings such as nuclear power, shipping and the military (Figure 21.2).

Notwithstanding convincing evidence from these high risk, safety critical occupations, the medical profession was slow to adopt non-technical skills training. Within the United Kingdom it is estimated that 10% of hospital patients will suffer an adverse event per annum of which 80% are attributable to human factors, which amounts to approximately 800 000 patients each year. Anaesthesia was the first medical specialty to truly embrace non-technical skills training (Fletcher et al., 2002). In the 1990s, driven by rising concerns over patient safety, the aviation CRM modules were adapted to produce an 'anaesthesia crisis resource management' course. There is an increasing body of evidence supporting the correlation between good non-technical skills and high standards of clinical care, as well as improved patient outcomes. Human factors training has since been incorporated into the education programmes for other medical specialties such as surgery, intensive care and emergency medicine (Brindley & Reynolds, 2011).

Developing a taxonomy

In 2003 a group of anaesthetists and psychologists developed a taxonomy of non-technical skills required for effective and safe anaesthetic practice within the operating theatre. The so-called anaesthetists' non-technical skills (ANTS) system distinguishes between four fundamental categories, notably the cognitive domains of situational awareness, decision making and task management, and the interpersonal domain of team working (Patey et al., 2005). As outlined in Figure 21.3 each of these four core elements can be further subdivided into 'skill elements', thus providing a framework through which anaesthetists can identify and assess non-technical skills in their colleagues, as well as reflect on their own behaviour. Although the ability to cope with fatigue and stress are not described separately their huge influence on each of the four categories is acknowledged. The utility of the ANTS taxonomy is not restricted to the field of anaesthesia because the skills identified are transferable across professional boundaries both within and outwith medicine.

Situational awareness

In its simplest form situational awareness (SA) is an appreciation of one's surroundings. It refers to an individual's ability to perceive environmental elements, comprehend their meaning and use this information to predict future events (Figure 21.4) taking account of the time available until a critical event takes place, or alternatively until an intervention is required. Since one's environment is constantly changing, SA is a dynamic process which relies upon excellent attention and a good working memory. However, it is well recognised that long-term memory has a role to play in SA, particularly when the limitations of human attention and working memory are exposed in times of stress or information overload. An example of good SA in the healthcare professions is the paramedic who checks that it is safe to approach a trauma victim in a potentially hazardous environment to avoid sustaining an injury themselves.

Decision making

Decision making describes the process of selecting a course of action from a variety of available options using a combination of past experiences and new information. Like SA it is a dynamic construct because one must constantly re-evaluate in light of the outcomes of one's decisions. Good decision making depends upon good SA but the two skills are discrete concepts and it is possible for an individual to correctly gather information, synthesise it and anticipate future events yet make poor decisions. Imagine if the paramedic in the earlier example accurately identifies environmental dangers yet attempts to resuscitate the patient when it is unsafe to do so, resulting in an injury to themself and ultimately delaying the patient's treatment. This highlights the importance of balancing risk in decision making.

Task management

This involves the utilisation of available resources to achieve goals whilst ensuring that work is planned and prioritised appropriately and performed to the highest standards.

Team working

Team working describes the skill set required to function in a group context to achieve task completion, and relies upon excellent communication skills in addition to the reciprocal qualities of leadership and followership. A team of experts does not necessarily constitute an expert team and within medicine there is now a greater focus on team training, particularly in an interprofessional setting, to improve patient outcomes.

Simulation provides excellent opportunities for the learning and assessment of all these non-technical skills if participants and teams can accept the 'fiction contract' and immerse themselves in the scenarios.

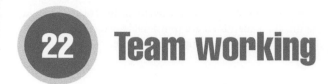

22 Team working

Figure 22.1 The five dimensions of teamwork and enabling mechanisms. Source: Salas et al., 2005. Reproduced with permission of SAGE Publications.

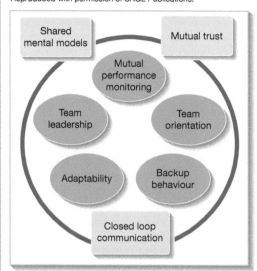

Box 22.1 An approach to simulation-based team training.

Course design
- Involve participants in course development
- Base learning objectives on theoretical models of teamwork
- Clearly define the learning outcomes and make them explicit to participants
- Consider learner level and match with task difficulty

Learning approaches
- The course and instructors should model good teamwork principles
- Use a mix of learning approaches, e.g. simulations, videos, didactic sessions

Simulations
- Familiarise learners with the simulation environment
- Explicitly state rules and processes
- Aim to trigger the thinking and behaviours involved in teamwork in the clinical environment
- Ensure the simulation is designed to meet the learning objectives
- Include a range of complexity, environments and teamwork challenges

Debriefing
- Use a structured model for feedback, e.g. attend to feelings; clarify what happened; explore why it happened, the results of certain behaviors, and how things could be done differently; identify lessons for future clinical practice
- Use a teamwork measurement instrument to facilitate feedback

Programme evaluation
- Evaluate retention of learning after 3–6 months
- Seek evidence for transfer of learning to clinical practice

Table 22.1 Part of a team measurement instrument. Source: Adapted from Weller et al., 2011.

A leader was clearly established	Excellent: One person centralised information and decision making and coordinated the actions of the team Poor: Unclear who was taking the lead, information not centralised, action of individuals not coordinated
The leader maintained an overview of the situation	Excellent: Kept on top of all the information available, and how tasks were being implemented Poor: Leader slow to notice new information, failed to notice that some tasks were not being done
Each team member had a clear role	Excellent: Leader explicitly designated all roles to team members Poor: No role designation, some roles unassigned, unclear what role each team member had
The leader's instructions were explicit	Excellent: Instructions were clearly audible, easy to understand, with sufficient detail to avoid confusion Poor: Unclear, inaudible, or imprecise instructions, e.g. 'give some adrenaline'
The leader's verbal instructions and verbal communications were directed	Excellent: Used person's name when giving instruction Poor: Use of 'someone', no indication of who the communication was meant for
When team members received instructions they closed the communication loop	Excellent: For critical instructions, team members repeated it back for confirmation Poor: No acknowledgement that the instruction had been heard or would be acted upon
The leader's plan for treatment was communicated to the team	Excellent: Team members informed of the plan in sufficient detail for them to understand what was required Poor: No treatment plan was shared by the leader with the team
Priorities and orders of actions were communicated to the team	Excellent: When more than one task was needed at any time, the leader clarified what was most important Poor: Leader issued multiple requests without prioritising
The leader verbalised to the team possible future developments or requirements	Excellent: Leader anticipated and verbalised potential future development and what might be required Poor: Leader failed to inform team members of possible developments they could be preparing for
The team leader responded appropriately to queries from team members	Excellent: Input invited. Gave explanation or clarification in response to questioning from team members Poor: Input not invited or discouraged. Ignored or dismissed questions or concerns from team members
When the leader did not respond to concerns raised by team members, they persisted in seeking a response	Did this occur? Yes / No. If yes, Excellent: Team member persisted with concern until it was resolved Poor: Team member did not pursue their concern, and the issue remained unresolved
The leader verbalised important clinical interventions to the team	Excellent: Leader always / almost always told the team what s/he was doing and what was happening Poor: Leader rarely or never told the team what s/he was doing, or what was happening
Team members verbalised their clinical actions to the leader	Excellent: Team members consistently informed the leader when they were doing critical tasks Poor: Team members rarely or never told the team leader what they were doing
Global behavioural performance	Overall impression of the team performance

Healthcare Simulation at a Glance. First Edition. Kirsty Forrest and Judy McKimm. © 2019 John Wiley & Sons, Ltd.
Published 2019 by John Wiley & Sons, Ltd.

A team can be defined as two or more individuals, each with specific roles, working together towards a common goal. Collaborative practice in teams involves communication, sharing of information and joint problem solving and decision making between the members of the healthcare team as peers. It implies a shared responsibility and accountability of the team leader and every member of the team for patient care. Simulation provides an excellent means of helping existing teams work more effectively together, and of facilitating team working and collaboration with learners.

Importance of teamwork and collaborative practice

Modern healthcare is increasingly being delivered by teams of health professionals, and the ability to work in a team is now an essential competency for all health professionals. Failures in teamwork and communication make a substantial contribution to adverse events which affect between 6% and 16% of hospitalised patients. Observational studies document high rates of teamwork failures affecting patient outcomes.

Team training appears to be effective in other industries. A meta-analysis of studies of 2650 non-clinical teams improved team processes and outcomes when team members had participated in team training (Salas et al., 2005). In the operating room, better team communication is associated with a reduction in adverse events (Mazzocco et al., 2009), and reduced perioperative morbidity and mortality has been attributed to the introduction of the World Health Organisation surgical safety checklist, which was designed to improve teamwork (World Alliance for Patient Safety, 2008).

Team training and simulation

Simulation is an ideal educational approach to team training. Simulation can recreate the tasks and complexity of the clinical environment, but in a controlled manner, allowing manipulation and enhancement of the clinical experience to address the behaviours and attitudes which underpin effective teamwork. Simulation-based team training allows learners to engage in the dynamic processes of teamwork enhanced by structured, facilitated reflection on the experience during debriefing. In situ simulation adds a further dimension to team training. Teams work together in the environment in which they usually work, and simulation can identify other influences on team performance including organisational structures, resources, equipment and workspace design.

A useful theoretical model for team training describes five dimensions of teamwork and three underpinning mechanisms (Figure 22.1) (Salas et al., 2005). The important dimensions of team behaviour are:

1 Team leadership (plan and prioritise, coordinate, monitor team performance, and develop the team and establish a positive atmosphere).
2 Mutual performance monitoring (monitor teammates' performance).
3 Back-up behaviour (anticipate other team members' needs and shift workload).

4 Adaptability (adjust strategies, course of action or task allocation when the situation changes).
5 Team orientation (awareness of behaviours of others in the team, belief in team versus individual).

These five dimensions of teamwork behaviours are dependent on three coordinating, or enabling, mechanisms:
1 Mutual trust (shared belief that team members will perform their roles).
2 Shared mental models (common understanding of the goal, plan, tasks and roles).
3 Closed loop communication (information exchange directed from a sender to a receiver and confirmed by the receiver).

Designing simulation-based team training

Some useful strategies for designing simulation-based team training are shown in Box 22.1. A useful starting point is to engage potential learners in a needs analysis to identify the particular issues around teamwork and communication in their environment, and identify examples from their own experience on which to base simulations. A single simulation session on teamwork is unlikely to be effective by itself. Team training should be ongoing and integrated into other educational programmes, be they undergraduate or continuing professional development. Training of instructors is essential, and should encompass teamwork theory, interprofessional learning and simulation-based education.

As stated in Box 22.1, a teamwork measurement instrument can guide reflection on the simulation during debriefing, evaluate the effectiveness of training initiatives and measure progress. The items in such a measurement tool should be observable, easy to interpret and be supported by descriptors of good and poor performance. Part of an example of a teamwork measurement instrument is provided in Table 22.1 (Weller et al., 2011).

Interprofessional team working

The training of healthcare professionals has traditionally focused on the knowledge and skills of individual clinical practitioners. This has reinforced professional silos, and limited the ease with which health professionals can form effective teams. For example, a lack of understanding of others' roles and capabilities provides a challenge to the development of a shared mental model, ability to monitor team member performance and provide support. Progress towards a culture of teamwork and interdependence between the professions is hampered by the complexity of interprofessional relationships, entrenched individualism, lack of application of the safety lessons from other complex organisations, hierarchical structures and diffuse accountability.

Simulation provides a platform for interdisciplinary teams to work together on relevant clinical tasks to develop and practise a range of teamwork behaviours. During the facilitated debrief, participants can explore the roles and capabilities of other team members, expose assumptions, for example, about what information should be shared, and when to speak up, and explore attitudes towards leadership and shared decision making. As such, simulation can be a powerful vehicle for change.

23 Crisis management

Figure 23.1 Simulation training.

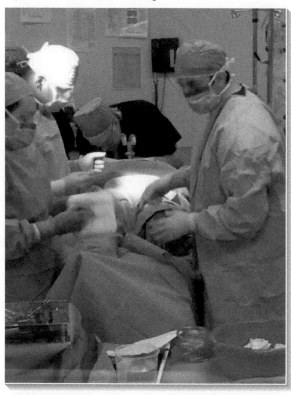

Box 23.1 Crisis preparation and avoidance.

Establish a team climate
- Build teamwork skills, climate of open communication and shared decision making

Develop communication and leadership skills
- In normal clinical contexts

Rehearse for crises
- Simulation training, mental rehearsal

Knowing and optimising the environment
- Cognitive aids for crises
- Know how to get help
- Know the names of team members

Anticipation and planning
- Briefing to establish shared team mental model
- Contingency planning for possible future events
- Advance preparation for periods of high workload

Box 23.2 Situational awareness.

Perception
- Gathering information (patient, monitors, team, environment)

Comprehension
- What does the information mean? What is the situation?

Prediction
- Where is this situation heading, what may happen next?

Box 23.3 Cognitive errors in a crisis.

Errors due to inattention (correct assessment, error in execution)
- Slip – automated actions without conscious control, e.g. drug administration error
- Lapse – omitting planned action, place-losing, forgetting intentions, e.g. forgetting to give drug planned for future time

Errors due to inadequate situational awareness (perception, comprehension, prediction)
- Inadequate knowledge (inexperience, junior staff), failure to appreciate complexity of the problem
- Fixation error – ignoring contradictory information, failing to consider alternatives, failure to predict what will happen next, e.g. 'this and only this', 'everything but this', 'everything's alright'
- Frequency gambling – going for the diagnosis based on the ease with which occurrences of similar events can be brought to mind (recent, frequent), without considering options
- Representativeness – going for the diagnosis based on similarity with common condition without close analysis

Box 23.4 Leadership style.

Democratic
- Collaborative leader, decisions made following discussion, compromises made, utilises all cognitive resources of team, may be too time consuming when rapid action required

Integrative
- Switch between collaborative and authoritarian depending on situational requirements but open to feedback or new information

Authoritarian
- Autocratic leader, makes decisions alone, input from team discouraged. Allows rapid action, but relies on leader being correct. Limited information sharing will limit ability of team to anticipate and thus support the leader or other team members

Healthcare Simulation at a Glance. First Edition. Kirsty Forrest and Judy McKimm. © 2019 John Wiley & Sons, Ltd.
Published 2019 by John Wiley & Sons, Ltd.

A crisis is any event that creates, or may lead to, an unstable or dangerous situation. Characteristically, crises are unexpected, non-routine events that create a high level of uncertainty and perceived threat, requiring immediate action to prevent a bad outcome.

Preparing for crises and crisis avoidance

Managing a crisis, or better still, avoiding a crisis, requires clinical expertise, excellent leadership skills and highly developed teamwork (see Chapter 22). Preparation for crises requires advanced clinical knowledge, clinical and teamwork skills and prior development of a team that can work together effectively under pressure (Box 23.1). Simulation-based training (Figure 23.1) is an excellent method for rehearsing for anticipated clinical crises (e.g. management of cardiac arrest, a woman bleeding heavily during delivery) (Goldstein, 2005) and developing skills in communication, collaboration, leadership and teamwork.

Simulation can also be used for large-scale simulations of 'disasters' by existing organisations and teams (e.g. terrorist attacks, infection outbreak) and in interprofessional learning at undergraduate or postgraduate levels (Livingston et al., 2016).

The sections that follow apply both to the management of a 'real' crisis and as a template for the rehearsal of a crisis through simulation.

Key activities of crisis management

When faced with a crisis, the tasks of the leader and the team are firstly to undertake an analysis of the situation, gathering relevant information to build a mental model of the situation. The next requirement is to plan the course of action which encompasses forming goals, assessing risks of different options, planning for action, prioritising tasks and making decisions. Execution of the planned tasks follows. Re-evaluation of the effects of the actions and the plan completes the cycle (Reason, 1990; Gaba et al., 1994).

Situational awareness

Situational awareness is the perception of information from the environment, the comprehension of what that information means, and the prediction of what may happen next (Box 23.2). Situational awareness is the basis of the mental model underpinning the decisions on patient management and can be prone to errors.

Effects of a crisis on thinking

A crisis typically evokes stress because of uncertain or ambiguous information, an unclear problem, time pressure to avert patient harm, or emotional response to perceived failure of care. In the stress created by a crisis, there can be a loss of situational awareness due to irrational or narrow thinking (failure to perceive all relevant information), disorganised problem solving and prioritisation (failure to comprehend the situation), focus on a single problem and failure to predict where the situation is heading.

Faced with a crisis, clinicians tend to reduce communication to the rest of the team – referred to as 'leader goes solo'. The team is left in a position of being unable to assist as the leader has not shared situational information. Due to the effects of stress, time pressure and cognitive overload, errors are likely to occur, as outlined in Box 23.3. Errors can create more stress and thus a vicious cycle of stress and error.

Error countermeasures

Expect errors to occur. Actively seek contradictions to the mental model and use the team to seek feedback on the mental model. Monitor team performance and point out mistakes of others: say what you noticed, express your concern and offer a solution. Wipe the slate clean – stand back, scan, reconsider, critically re-evaluate. Use cognitive aids when available. Seek help. Aim for hands-off leadership. The leader needs to focus on problem solving and on managing the tasks – to do this properly they cannot also be doing a task.

Leadership style in a crisis

Leadership styles in clinical teams range from democratic, where all are issues of patient care are discussed and decisions are made together, to authoritarian, where the leader makes decisions and the rest of the team carry out orders. There is a time and place for both styles depending on the situation. Democracy can be too slow in a rapidly evolving crisis. Successful authoritarian leadership depends a great deal on the leader being correct, and also being credible as the leader for the situation (Box 23.4). Leadership and followership can shift between individuals, depending on the situation and expertise of those involved. If time allows, a compromise would be to regularly invite feedback and situational information from the team.

Communication in a crisis

Effective communication is essential in a crisis to ensure accurate and timely task execution, and to develop a shared mental model of the situation.

Closed loop communication entails clear, concise and directed communication by the sender to the receiver, and acknowledgement by the receiver that the message has been heard and accurately interpreted. ISBAR is a commonly used structure for conveying information (I = identify self, S = state the situation, B = background, A = assessment of the situation, and R = request/recommendation).

Developing a shared mental model ensures team members are: working towards a common goal; understand tasks and priorities; can predict what the leader and other team members will require next, plan for it and provide support; and can contribute to problem solving and point out potential errors (St Pierre et al., 2008). The leader can develop a shared mental model through briefings and regular situation updates.

24 Simulated and standardised patients

Figure 24.1 Simulation activity.

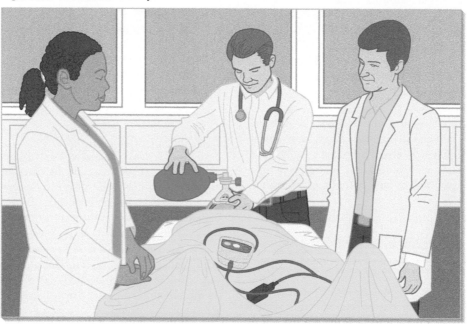

Box 24.1 Standardised/simulated patient definition. Source: SIRC, 2019.

Standardised/simulated patients are individuals who are trained to portray a patient with a specific condition in a realistic, standardised and repeatable way (where portrayal/presentation varies based only on learner performance). SPs can be used for teaching and assessment of learners including but not limited to history/consultation, physical examination and other clinical skills in simulated clinical environments. SPs can also be used to give feedback and evaluate student performance.

Box 24.2 Examples of educational or other activities where SPs have been used successfully. Source: Forrest et al. 2013. Reproduced with permission of John Wiley and Sons.

Communication skills
- Taking a patient history
- Gaining consent for procedures or surgery
- Handling difficult conversations, such as breaking bad news, being open about an error, discussing wishes about end of life
- Developing advanced consultation skills
- Undertaking telephone interviews
- Using structured communication tools, e.g. for escalating care in acute emergencies
- As part of a hybrid simulation exercise in order to explore the influence of context on ability to communicate effectively

Physical examinations
- Teaching physical examination skills with normal signs
- Developing ability to display (simulate) abnormal signs
- Portraying patients with acutely abnormal physiology (usually aided by moulage)
- Performing as a specialist teaching associate to help teach intimate examinations

Evaluating clinical services
- Acting as a 'mystery shopper' to assess performance of community- or hospital-based patient services and clinics

The inclusion of simulated patients (SPs) has grown over the past 50 years in the context of training and assessment of clinical skills in healthcare professionals (Figure 24.1). This has been driven by a growing recognition of the educational advantages offered by this methodology, as well as responding to the changing landscape and constraints being faced in clinical education including workforce development, healthcare delivery and the expectations of patients and the public regarding the safety and quality of care.

Definitions

The terms 'simulated patient' and 'standardised patient' are often used interchangeably, the latter being more commonly used in

Healthcare Simulation at a Glance. First Edition. Kirsty Forrest and Judy McKimm. © 2019 John Wiley & Sons, Ltd.
Published 2019 by John Wiley & Sons, Ltd.

the North American literature. Other terms include role player, medical actor, simulator, clinical teaching associate, patient educator (instructor) or patient expert (Box 24.1).

Barrows (1993) defined the terms as:

- **Simulated patient**: someone who has been coached or trained to portray a specific patient when given a history and physical examination, incorporating a display of relevant symptoms, signs, emotions and behaviour.
- **Standardised patient**: also includes real patients who have been coached to present *their own illness* (e.g. a heart murmur or signs of a stroke) in a standardised way.

History

Howard Barrows (an American neurologist and academic) pioneered the concept of simulated patients in the 1960s (Barrows & Abrahamson, 1964) based on several sentinel experiences in his career:

- Observing medical students 'carrying out their professional tasks', addressing errors and improving their history taking, physical examination and 'thinking' skills, as well as overcoming the time-consuming nature of learning.
- Discovering that a patient selected for specialty training summative exams in neurology deliberately altered presentation of his physical signs to one learner who he had felt was 'hostile and performing a very uncomfortable examination', thus influencing the outcome of this assessment.
- Training a lay person to simulate a range of physical neurological signs, anxieties and concerns based on the emotional component of the disease process. Using a checklist, the SP provided feedback following all encounters, including some unique insights into 'interpersonal skills' and 'thinking skills'.

The popularity of SPs grew slowly, however the widespread uptake of the objective structured clinical examination (OSCE) from the 1970s (Harden, 1975) led to a dramatic increase in demand for SPs who were trained to support OSCEs, particularly at the undergraduate level.

Learning and teaching

SPs have been included in the teaching and assessment of practical skills, in particular the integrated teaching of technical and communications skills in performing specific clinical procedures (Kneebone et al., 2002; Ker, 2003). Specialised examples of SP practice emerged, such as female SPs specifically trained to help teach undergraduate medical students, GP trainees, nurses and other health professionals. These include gynaecology teaching associates (GTAs) who are trained women who support students in learning to perform speculum and bimanual examinations by acting as an SP and teacher (Pickard et al., 2003). SPs can also be instructors in their own right (Nestel et al., 2002). Some SPs take part in hybrid simulations where a part task trainer is used in conjunction with an SP. The SP can then give feedback on the learner's communication skills, touch and pressure, and other non-technical skills. Trained SPs also support formative and summative assessment, providing instant feedback to learners, particularly in clinical competence (e.g. in OSCEs) and also in selection processes (Box 24.2).

Advantages of SPs

The advantages of SPs for teaching and assessing include:

- *Availability and planning*: SPs overcome the uncertainty of relying on the availability of suitable patients.
- *Consistency*: the same SP for several students consecutively with presentations staying the same.

- *Safe teaching environment*: SPs allow students to practise dealing with problems which, if handled inexpertly, could be very distressing or damaging for real patients, e.g. bereavement or breaking bad news.
- *Direct feedback*: SPs can provide timely, constructive and honest feedback to the student from the patient's perspective, either 'in role' or 'out of role', during a 'time out' period mid-scenario, or at the end of the exercise.
- *Deliberate practice*: the opportunity to repeat consultations or examinations and try different approaches offers learners a unique opportunity to refine skills and competences or apply skills under increasingly complex contexts, e.g. hybrid practical simulations combining a part task trainer and a SP.
- *Reducing clinical educator requirements*: some SPs are trained in high level facilitation skills and act as clinical educators within well-rehearsed educational activities or summative assessments.

Disadvantages of SPs

The disadvantages of SPs for teaching and assessing include the following:

- It is time consuming to recruit, train and organise SPs.
- SPs cannot completely duplicate the 'real' patient.
- Some conditions are not easily assessed through simulation, e.g. the physical signs of oedema or stroke.

Selection and training

Educational institutions use local advertisement campaigns (Collins & Harden, 1998), word of mouth, the internet and SP agencies to recruit and select SPs.

Selection criteria should include the following:

- The requirement for the SP to perform under varying conditions and contexts, and with different levels of responsibility for contributing actively to feedback.
- Broader professional behaviours, attitudes and perspectives of the prospective SP toward healthcare, the system(s) in which it is organised and delivered, and toward the professionals (or students) who they will meet as part of their role.
- Negative attitudes or deeply held beliefs should preclude selection.
- SPs should be representative of the patient population they are asked to embody.

Particular difficulties arise in recruiting for some cultural or age-related (e.g. paediatric) groups, and those with learning or physical disabilities. Some institutions employ professional actors as SPs, especially where patient portrayals might require simulation of physical findings or be highly emotionally charged. For less complex scenarios willing, 'healthy' volunteers from many walks of life (including students) can fulfil the role. Medical student participation can provide a unique insight into the patients' perspectives on consultations which may help them become better doctors, develop their teaching skills and act as positive role models.

SPs should be trained to work in the context in which they are required and preferably trained by clinical teachers if they are to be involved in clinical skills education or assessment. Typically, SPs are trained in history and consultation; to portray physical signs; to portray mental health issues; to provide feedback; to facilitate small groups; and to act as patient educators. Many resources exist to help organisations develop SPs in their different roles. For example, the simulated patient network http://www.simulatedpatientnetwork.org, which includes information on standards of best practice (Lewis et al., 2017).

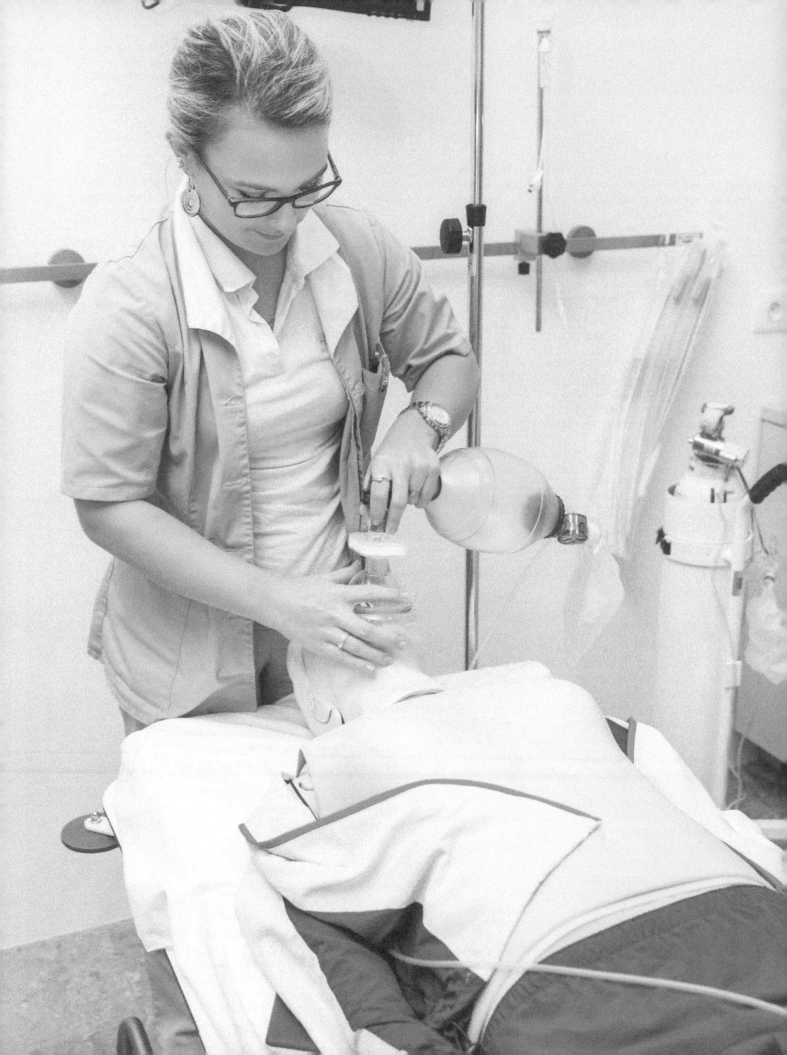

Assessment, feedback and remediation

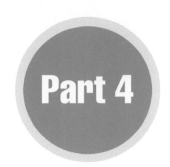

Part 4

Chapters

25 Principles of assessment

Practice points

- Simulations are a useful adjunct to assessment processes, especially for practical skills and procedures, and for some non-technical skills
- Performance in a simulation can be measured through technical means but human judgement is required for more complex encounters
- Rating instruments comprise checklists (list of observable actions) and global rating scales (generic level of performance)

Figure 25.1 Miller's pyramid with examples of assessment modalities at each level. WPBA, workplace-based assessment; SP, standardised patient; OSCE, objective structured clinical examination; CbD, case-based discussion; MCQ, multiple choice question; SAQ, short answer question.

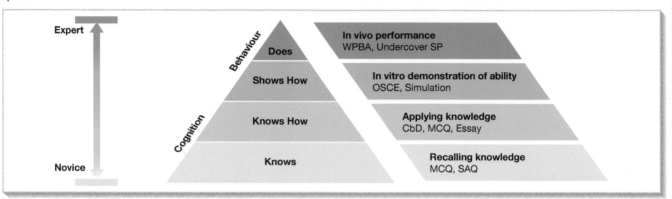

Figure 25.2 High fidelity mannequins have not replaced the need for human assessors – yet!.

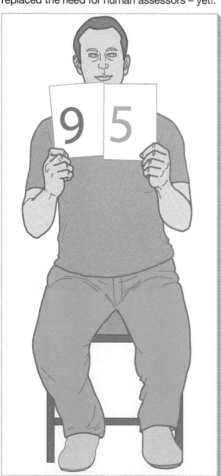

Figure 25.3 Flowchart for the development of a simulation-based assessment.

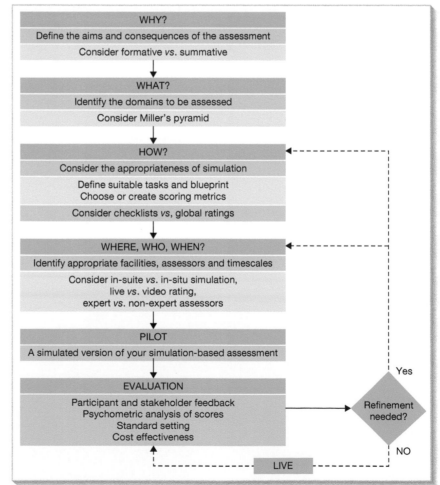

Healthcare Simulation at a Glance. First Edition. Kirsty Forrest and Judy McKimm. © 2019 John Wiley & Sons, Ltd.
Published 2019 by John Wiley & Sons, Ltd.

Assessment drives learning and is therefore integral to any educational programme. The assessment of learners in health professions' education has three main aims.

1 Identify learning needs in order to drive future learning.

2 Safeguard patients and reassure the public by ensuring that learners meet professional standards.

3 Rank applicants for recruitment to postgraduate training programmes and jobs (Epstein, 2007).

Assessments designed to fulfil the first aim are described as *formative* while those meeting the latter aims are described as *summative*.

What to assess?

Healthcare practice is complex and requires proficiency across the three main domains of learning: cognitive (knowledge), psychomotor (skills) and affective (behaviours) domains. Because of its closeness to 'what practitioners do in the workplace', simulation offers scope for assessing learner proficiency in all of these domains. For example, a team-based cardiac arrest scenario could simultaneously assess clinical diagnostic skills, ability to coordinate and perform cardiopulmonary resuscitation and interpersonal communication. Trying to assess too much within a short time frame however, risks overloading the assessors and hence reducing the validity of the assessment.

Miller's pyramid offers a framework for analysing different levels of assessment, from pure knowledge at its base to complex behaviours in practice at the apex (Figure 25.1) (Miller, 1990). Simulation-based assessment sits mainly in the 'shows how' level but modalities such as 'undercover patients or secret shoppers' and in situ simulation edge into the 'does' level. While less 'authentic' than workplace-based assessment, simulation offers greater standardisation (all learners assessed in the same way), reliability (assessment scores are repeatable) and the opportunity for learners to be assessed without compromising patient safety.

How to measure performance?

Simulation is not the ideal vehicle for all types of assessment and the decision to assess learner achievement via simulation requires careful consideration. Basic science or clinical knowledge, for example, is more readily and cheaply assessed by multiple choice tests. The constructs to be measured (e.g. suturing skill, patient empathy) need to be carefully mapped (blueprinted) to the simulated tasks through which they will be assessed. Thought must also be given to the appropriate level of fidelity needed for an assessment. Why use a full manikin when a plastic arm will do?

Assessee performance in a simulation can be measured in two ways. Technical measures captured by equipment in the simulation suite (e.g. motion times, path lengths, ventilation rates) are increasingly available but their scope is largely restricted to the psychomotor domain. Assessment of the more complex human dimensions of the clinical encounter requires human judgement and the use of reliable rating instruments (Figure 25.2).

Rating instruments fall broadly into two types: checklists and global rating scales. A checklist comprises a list of observable actions, usually scored on a yes/no basis according to whether or not they were performed by the assessee. A global rating scale comprises an ordered list of levels of performance to which numerical scores are attributed. Generic scales (e.g. 1 = poor, 2 = borderline, 3 = satisfactory, 4 = excellent) are frequently used because the same scale can be applied to many different constructs.

Who should rate performance?

Learners in healthcare may be assessed by practitioners (experts or higher level trainees), patients (real, simulated or standardised), their peers or themselves. Rater choice will be guided by the required level of expertise, the need for training/benchmarking, cost, availability and the consequences of the assessment. For example, a high stakes professional examination would demand more experienced assessors than a basic life support assessment for undergraduate students. Assessors can be passive observers or, as in the case of patient assessors, may actively participate in the simulation.

Where to assess?

In situ simulation can offer greater authenticity and other advantages over in suite simulation (see Chapter 20). Because of limitations on the availability of 'live' facilities and the need for standardisation of assessee experience, however, its use in assessment may be restricted to situations where assessee numbers are small. Simple classroom-type facilities on the other hand, can and should be used in preference to expensive simulation suites for low fidelity simulations.

When to assess?

Traditionally, judgement takes place during, or shortly following, task performance. The video equipment in modern simulation facilities, however, opens the door to asynchronous assessment of videoed performance by multiple judges using multiple rating tools. Video can also enhance learner feedback (debriefing) and facilitate assessment and training of assessors. These advantages must be weighed against the fact that the video cannot capture everything that happens.

Evaluation

Good quality assessments should exhibit strengths in the following areas:

• *Acceptability*: the assessment is seen as fair and appropriate by stakeholders (learners, faculty, institutions, the public).

• *Reliability*: the assessment would produce similar scores if conducted in similar circumstances, such as on other occasions or using other raters or scenarios.

• *Validity*: confidence can be placed in the meaning of the assessment scores (e.g. that the learner has mastered a particular skill or is a 'competent' health professional) (Cook & Hatala, 2016).

• *Educational impact*: feedback on the learner's performance, guides and stimulates future learning.

• *Feasibility*: setting up and running the assessment is logistically possible and practicable.

• *Cost efficiency*: the consequences of the assessment represent good value in relation to the time, money and resources (both human and technological) put into it (PMETB, 2007).

Figure 25.3 summarises the stages for the development of a simulation-based assessment.

26 Learner-centred assessment

Figure 26.1 Simulation effectiveness: skills acquisition curve showing the impact of zero risk training.

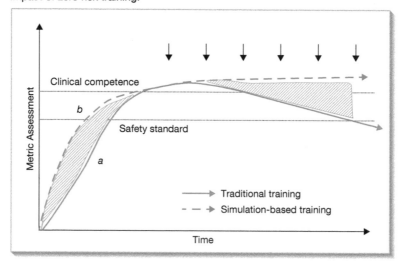

Figure 26.2 Some learner-focused simulation activities such as (a) nurses with a paediatric simulator and (b) learners with an adult simulator.

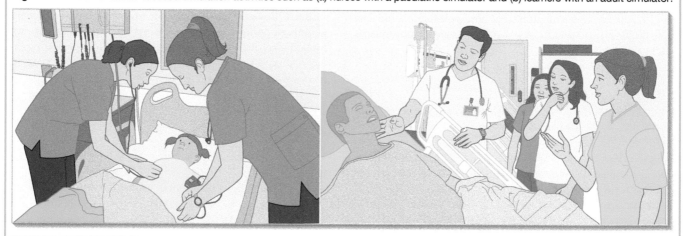

Healthcare Simulation at a Glance. First Edition. Kirsty Forrest and Judy McKimm. © 2019 John Wiley & Sons, Ltd.
Published 2019 by John Wiley & Sons, Ltd.

earner-centred assessments can be targeted at learning that participants and faculty actually want to achieve, and shifts the focus of educational interventions from *teaching* to *learning* (Huba & Freed, 2000). In this way assessments can be designed so that they are more meaningful to learners taking part in simulation at various stages of their training. Assessments within a curriculum or educational programme should be mapped to defined learning outcomes which are appropriate for learners at that particular stage of training. These learning outcomes are integrated into national curriculum documents at both undergraduate and postgraduate levels. Within each curriculum, certain learning outcomes will lend themselves more readily for assessment using simulation.

Competency-based medical education

The concept of competency-based medical education (CBME) promotes learner centredness and focuses on the outcomes of an educational programme and the abilities of the learner that define competence (Frank et al., 2010). Clearly defined competences provide explicit goals for the learner and milestones that individuals can target for their own learning. CBME de-emphasises assessment of knowledge in favour of skills and behaviours which can be assessed with observable competencies. CBME can encourage learners to track their own progress between milestones which may be achieved at different rates. Once competencies and milestones have been mapped to a curriculum, educational methods including simulation can be developed along with assessment tools for the learner. Careful design of assessment tools is important to ensure that assessments are not seen as just a tick box exercise and result in meaningful judgements about performance and feedback that is useful to the trainee. Some programmes incorporate entrustable professional activities (EPAs) as units of assessment where learners are assessed on the level of supervision required to undertake a particular task. This type of assessment uses expert judgement to measure observed performance of clinical activities or simulations to identify levels of supervision required in the workplace.

Simulation and learner centredness

Simulation lends itself well for learners to demonstrate skills and attitudes through the use of part task trainers, simulated patients and team-based simulations, and can steepen the learning curve towards proficiency targets. Figure 26.1 shows how simulated practise can improve levels of performance and prevent skill decay once a level of competence has been achieved. This graph shows how skill acquisition progresses over time to defined targets, with traditional versus simulation training for procedural skills, such as central line insertion (Dong et al., 2010). Simulation-enhanced training (plot *b*) can lead to accelerated learning compared with traditional training (plot *a*). Repeated simulations (arrows on Figure 26.1), after proficiency has been achieved, maintain levels of capability and prevent skills decay, which can occur over time when there is no further clinical experience or opportunities for practise. Point of care simulations increase access and opportunities for learners to practise new skills on part task trainers at regular intervals.

Proficiency-based simulation allows learners to be assessed according to pre-set standards that need to be reached before they can progress to the next stage of the programme. Some training programmes assess skills in this way before trainees can perform surgery on real patients. Learners can practise their skills through self-directed learning on simulators. Depending on the skill being measured, assessments can utilise both videos and mechanical sensors incorporated within the simulators. Deliberate practise of psychomotor skills using simulation repetitively can aid mastery of learning for particular techniques.

Learner feedback

Best practice when utilising simulation involves providing feedback at every opportunity (McGaghie et al., 2010). Feedback should be provided during both formative and summative assessments in order to influence future learning and guide practice. Feedback for team-based simulations can involve learner-centred assessment during group debriefs if the debrief is conducted well. Debrief techniques such as advocacy inquiry, guided team self-correction and circular questioning promote learner and group reflection so that learner-centred assessments involve self-assessment and peer assessment as well as faculty assessment. Expertly facilitated debriefs involve low levels of facilitation in order to encourage reflection on behalf of the participants. For more detail on methods of debriefing, see Chapter 28.

Portfolios of learning

Portfolios allow the learner to collate a longitudinal record of evidence related to learning outcomes in a programme. This can involve assessments of clinical competences through simulations or workplace-based exercises (Figure 26.2), log-book data of the number of procedural skills, reflective accounts of clinical/simulated encounters and certification of relevant training/assessments undertaken. Portfolios help the learner to reflect on their own progress between milestones within a programme and aid meaningful discussion during appraisals with educational supervisors.

to patient safety, therefore remediation is a necessary part of the professional development cycle. If remediation does not have the desired improvement, then learners may have to repeat an element of their education or training or leave the course. Practitioners who fail to reach required professional standards may have their licence to practice revoked.

Approach and mind set

The first step is for the tutor or supervisor to work with each individual to discover what exactly is going on for that person. An individualised, personal approach seems to work best, particularly when a more complex intervention relating to the person's personality or communication skills is required (Cohen et al., 2014). The person involved needs to have enough self-insight to recognise they need to improve, as well as the motivation to engage in the remediation process. For most people, the primary motivation will be extrinsic (e.g. a needing to pass a high stakes examination or retain a licence) but intrinsic (internal) motivation is also needed to engage fully in the remediation, and the resilience to persevere when things are tough. Box 33.1 sets out the sequence of steps involved in remediation activities.

Role of simulation

Simulation is probably most useful to help with remediation in cases where a learner or practitioner has been identified (through formal assessment or clinical practice supervisor reports) as needing to improve their practical or procedural clinical skills or clinical reasoning, has not demonstrated a professional enough approach for their stage of training or practice, or has exhibited unprofessional behaviours (including poor communication skills).

Practical skills and competencies

Skills deficits are best remediated through deliberate, conscious, focused practise with feedback. Depending on the skill or competency involved, remediation might go right back to basics, e.g. watching a video or demonstration of a skill or procedure by an 'expert'. Typically, remediation will first involve being observed carrying out the skill or procedure by the teacher so that the specific deficiencies can be identified. From a patient safety perspective, using a simulator (if appropriate) rather than a real patient enables the learner to have more attempts at the procedure. The skill might be fairly simple, e.g. cannulation or catheterisation, or involve a more complex, higher risk procedure such as delivering a baby with an atypical presentation. The simulator must be chosen to enable the learner to demonstrate the skill as authentically as possible.

Simulators that provide haptic feedback can be useful for invasive procedures (such as those carried out in surgery) or palpation. They provide feedback on specific actions and motor skills through providing cutaneous and kinaesthetic information to the user. Many studies report that these simulators are highly effective in the development of such skills (e.g. Gottlieb et al., 2017; McGrath et al., 2018) although there is little in the literature concerning remediation specifically.

Clinical reasoning and decision-making

Simulation is also used to remediate for more complex skills such as critical thinking, clinical reasoning and clinical judgement (Evans & Harder, 2013; Rencic et al., 2016). Simulators

used to help develop such skills include computer-based 'virtual patients' or 'virtual scenarios' in which learners are required to make diagnoses, clinical judgements and decisions about referral and treatment options. Feedback is provided to the learner about their choices and decisions, a record is given to the teacher about decisions made, and clinical cases or scenarios of varying complexity can be used.

High fidelity manikins and virtual reality (VR) simulation can also help develop and remediate complex decision-making skills, particularly in acute, complex or emergency situations. Bond et al. (2008) suggest that simulation can help develop confidence and quicker, accurate decision making, develop competence in a range of procedures and situations, and develop situational awareness in a wider range of cases (including those infrequently found or extremely complex).

Human simulators (e.g. simulated or standardised patients) can also be used for more complex skills such as taking a history, clerking a patient, explaining treatment options or carrying out a physical or psychological examination. The 'patient' can provide feedback to the learner which, when coupled with that from an observer, can stimulate a detailed and comprehensive exploration of critical thinking, clinical reasoning and decision-making skills. Simulation can enable 'think aloud' verbal protocol analysis which may help to pinpoint and remediate the deficiencies in an individual's thought and reasoning processes (Bond et al., 2008).

Professionalism issues or concerns

Professionalism issues are best addressed through explicit instruction and demonstration, guided practice, mentored reflection, observation and interaction with role models (who can be 'real' or simulated, e.g. an actor). Whilst many of the simulation activities already described are also appropriate for remediating in the professionalism domain, simulation can provide additional assistance in areas such as team working, leadership and communication with patients, families and colleagues (Box 33.2).

Regan et al. (2016) describe a training and remediation programme in interpersonal and communication skills and professionalism for trainees with a simulation component. The programme is structured around key milestones, each of which has a remediation strategy. Simulated case scenarios help learners improve their cultural competency, humanism and compassion with patients; to utilise their strengths and understand their limitations; practice reflection; be open to receive feedback; and to deal with medical uncertainty.

Other activities such as multiprofessional case conferences, team-working tasks, leadership activities and conflict situations can all be simulated to help learners develop respect for others, to negotiate decisions and conflict, and to develop enhanced communication skills.

Summary

Simulation is a useful adjunct to other forms of remediation, but questions still remain about the transferability of learning through simulation to the real clinical environment and how we can best observe learners or practitioners when working with real patients with real-time service pressures. Whilst simulation must not be used as the only means of signing off complex communication skills, it certainly has a place in helping to provide a safe place for remediation through practice and feedback.

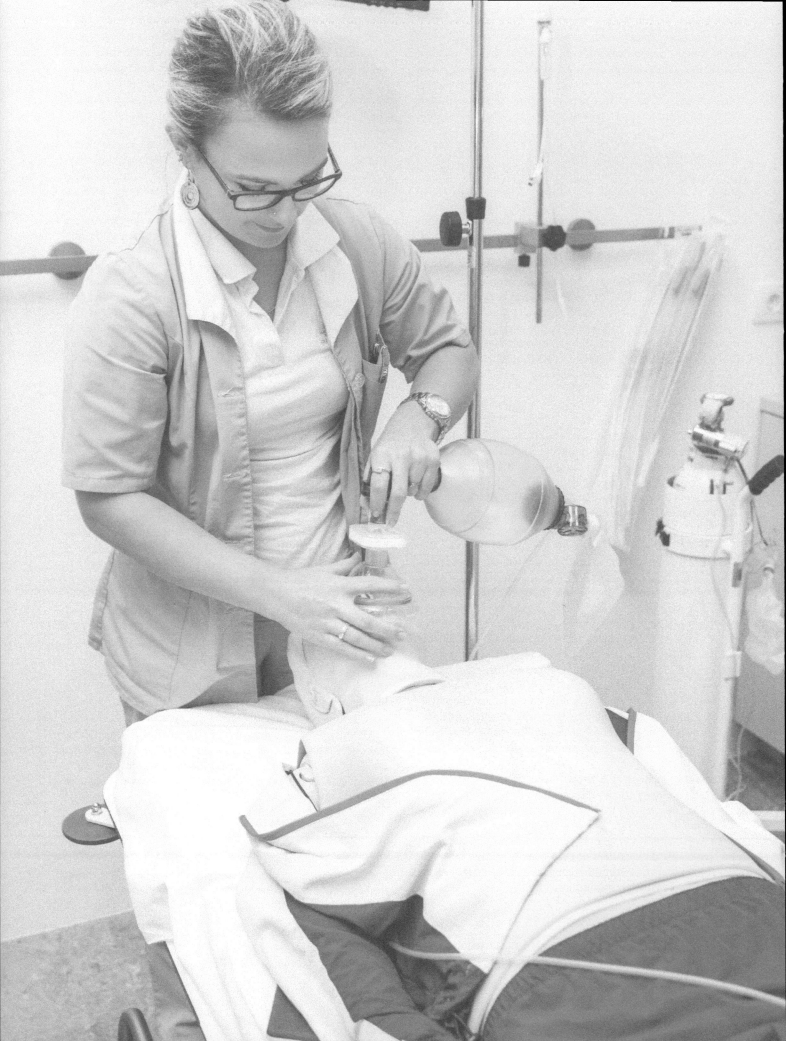

Developing your practice

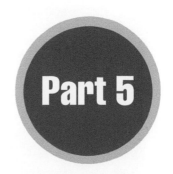

Part 5

Chapter

34 Developing your practice

Figure 34.1 Developing as a simulation educator. This model is adapted from McKimm et al. (2017) and indicates how educators might engage with different simulation activities along a continuum. It summarises some of the knowledge, skills and activities individuals might need to acquire and engage in as they develop their simulation educator practice.

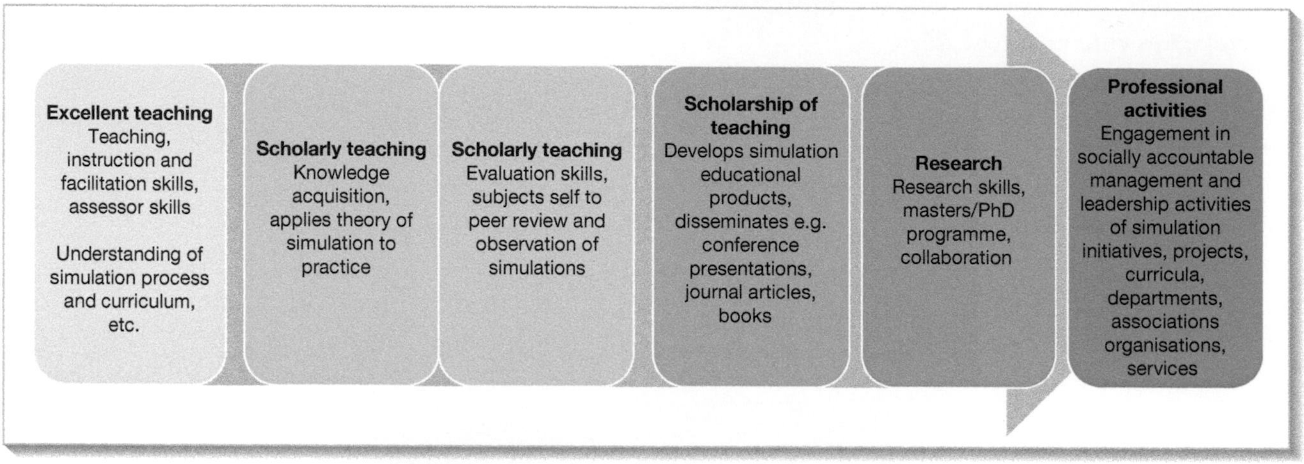

Excellent teaching
Teaching, instruction and facilitation skills, assessor skills

Understanding of simulation process and curriculum, etc.

Scholarly teaching
Knowledge acquisition, applies theory of simulation to practice

Scholarly teaching
Evaluation skills, subjects self to peer review and observation of simulations

Scholarship of teaching
Develops simulation educational products, disseminates e.g. conference presentations, journal articles, books

Research
Research skills, masters/PhD programme, collaboration

Professional activities
Engagement in socially accountable management and leadership activities of simulation initiatives, projects, curricula, departments, associations organisations, services

Figure 34.2 Simulation trainer.

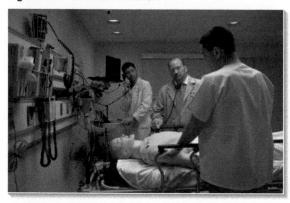

Figure 34.3 Conferences are useful for learning and disseminating knowledge.

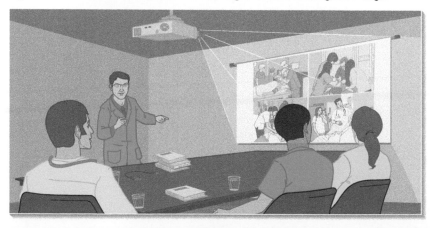

Healthcare Simulation at a Glance. First Edition. Kirsty Forrest and Judy McKimm. © 2019 John Wiley & Sons, Ltd.
Published 2019 by John Wiley & Sons, Ltd.

The education of health professionals is becoming increasingly professionalised and the opportunities for simulation education are increasing in scope as well as the technologies involved. As hospital wards and clinics become more crowded, the opportunities for learners to work with 'real' patients are becoming harder to manage. As we have seen throughout the book, there are many ways exist to utilise simulation in health professions' education and the academic or clinical teacher needs to be aware of these. In this chapter, we are not focusing on general applications of simulation (such as including role play in a classroom session) but on the educator who has a keen interest in simulation to help enhance the learning of clinical (technical and non-technical) skills.

Professional development in simulation education can be considered as running along a continuum from 'simply' being a teacher of a few simulation sessions, through to a leader or manager of a simulation programme or centre (Figure 34.1). Along the way, most educators develop their own scholarly practice, that is they become more aware of the theories of learning that underpin effective simulation education and, over time, might start to contribute towards the body of knowledge through conference presentations and publications. We will consider each of these 'steps' in turn.

Excellent teaching

Often the first step into teaching simulation activities is being involved in clinical skills teaching, with simulated patients, models or manikins, sometimes with whole body simulators (Figure 34.2). To become an excellent teacher, a variety of educational development activities exist which can be undertake alongside learning by working with and observing experienced teachers. Being able to ask questions and obtain feedback on your teaching practice is an excellent way to improve your teaching and many simulation activities are 'team taught', i.e. taught by more than one teacher, which facilitates professional conversations as you strive to improve the programme.

An obvious formal starting point to develop your practical teaching skills is to attend short courses and workshops, which may well be provided through the university or healthcare organisation for which you are working. Whilst these might not be specifically about simulation teaching, learning the fundamentals of small group teaching, setting learning outcomes, course planning and design, assessment and evaluation, will all be helpful. Some courses include observation of your teaching practice which, whilst it may seem daunting, can be very helpful.

Scholarly teaching

If you intend to become more regularly and formally involved in simulation education, then you need to develop your scholarly practice: practice grounded in theory (Bligh & Brice, 2009).

> Having a knowledge base and understanding of educational principles and terminology not only gives you more confidence and credibility in educational settings but also should help you to deliver high-quality education. (McKimm et al., 2017)

A scholarly practitioner understands the evidence behind why education and learning is being planned and delivered in the way it is and how to evaluate it, not just what is being taught and how to do it.

Keeping up to date with your subject and learning more can be achieved through reading journals and other publications and engagement with professional associations. This should be ongoing throughout your career. To develop as a scholarly practitioner, you will probably need to undertake a formal education programme. A range of postgraduate degree programmes are provided by universities and colleges (face to face and online), some of which offer specific degrees or modules in simulation education. Other programmes in simulation are provided by medical and health profession educational associations, such as the Association for simulated Practice in Healthcare (ASPiH, see http://aspih.org.uk), the Society for Simulation in Healthcare (SSH, see www.ssh.org) or An International Association for Medical Education (AMME, see https://amee.org). Institutional accreditation for education can also be sort from organisations such as the Society in Europe for Simulation Applied to Medicine (SESAM, see https://www.sesam-web.org/).

Scholarship of teaching

At this stage of the continuum, educators will be starting to think about how they can contribute to the body of knowledge about simulation education. One way is to develop simulation products or educational resources that can be shared with others. Another way is to disseminate your work through publications or presentations at conferences (Figure 34.3). In the early stages, it is likely that you will collaborate with other people to put posters about your work into local or national conferences, gradually building up to writing articles in newsletters or blogs, then to publishing books or articles in peer reviewed journals. Whilst general health professions' journals include publications on simulation activities, a few journals are devoted specifically to simulation (including in healthcare and education). These include *Simulation* (Sage Journals), *BMJ Simulation & Technology Enhanced Learning* (BMJ Journals) and *Advances in Simulation* (BioMed Central).

Research

Some educators will be actively engaged in simulation-based research (SBR) to improve the practice of simulation education. These might be large- or small-scale projects. They may be undertaken as part of a degree, through internally or externally funded initiatives, or simply because of a keen interest. Martin (2016) suggests that standardised guidelines are needed to ensure all simulation studies are performed to the highest standard, and a number of groups are actively working on developing reporting guidelines for SBR (Cheng et al., 2016; Sevdalis et al., 2016).

Professional activities

We mentioned conferences and meetings as opportunities for disseminating your work, but they are also vital venues for networking with like-minded people, learning about new developments and hearing from experts and people whose work you have read. Joining professional organisations often gives access to a range of educational resources, blogs, webinars and other activities. A number of associations now offer professional recognition for your educator role, including the Academy of Medical Educators (AoME), the Higher Education Academy (HEA) and AMEE.

As you become more expert yourself, you may well want to take a leadership or management role in your own organisation or programme, or in an external association. Offering to work on projects or initiatives is interesting in itself and also helps you gain experience and expertise in specific areas. If you start to move into a formal management, leadership or entrepreneurial role, then you may wish to undertake further professional development in these areas.

References

ACSQHC (Australian Commission on Safety and Quality in Health Care) (2011) *National Safety and Quality Health Service Standards.* http://www.safetyandquality.gov.au/wp-content/uploads/2011/09/NSQHS-Standards-Sept-2012.pdf (accessed February 2019).

Aggarwal R, Mytton OT, Debrew M et al. (2010) Training and simulation for patient safety. *Quality and Safety in Health Care,* 19(suppl 2), i34–43.

AHRQ (Agency for Healthcare Research and Quality) (2015) *Team-STEPPS.* Available at http://teamstepps.ahrq.gov/teamstepps/index.html (accessed February 2019).

Andreatta P, Saxton E, Thompson M, Annich G (2011) Simulation-based mock codes significantly correlate with improved pediatric cardiopulmonary arrest survival rates. *Pediatric Critical Care Medicine,* 12, 33–38.

Bandura A (1977) *Social Learning Theory.* Oxford: Prentice-Hall.

Bandura A (2001) Social cognitive theory: an agentic perspective. *Annual Review of Psychology,* 52(1), 1–26.

Bargh JA (1994) The four horsemen of automaticity: awareness, intention, efficiency, and control in social cognition. In: Wyer Jr RS, Srull TK (eds) *Handbook of Social Cognition,* 2nd edn. Hillsdale, NJ: Lawrence Erlbaum Associates.

Barrows H (1993) An overview of the uses of standardized patients for teaching and evaluating clinical skill. *Academic Medicine,* 68, 443–453.

Barrows H, Abrahamson S (1964) The programmed patient: a technique for appraising student performance in clinical neurology. *Journal of Medical Education,* 39, 802–805.

Battista A. (2017). An activity theory perspective of how scenario-based simulations support learning: a descriptive analysis. *Advances in Simulation,* 2(23).

Beaubien JM, Baker DP (2004) The use of simulation for training teamwork skills in health care: how low can you go? *Quality and Safety in Health Care,* 13, i51–i56.

Benishek L, Lazzara E, Gaught W, Arcaro L, Okuda Y, Salas E (2014) The Template of Events for Applied and Critical Healthcare Simulation (TEACH Sim): a tool for systematic simulation scenario design. *Simulation in Healthcare,* 10(1), 21–30.

Biggs J (1996) Enhancing teaching through constructive alignment. *Higher Education,* 32, 347–64.

Biggs J (2014) Constructive alignment in university teaching. *HERDSA Review of Higher Education,* 1, 5–22.

Bligh J, Brice J (2009) Further insights into the roles of the medical educator: the importance of scholarly management. *Academic Medicine,* 84, 1161–1165.

Bond W, Kuhn G, Binstadt E et al. (2008) The use of simulation in the development of individual cognitive expertise in emergency medicine. *Academic Emergency Medicine,* 15(11), 1037–1045.

Brewin J, Ahmed K, Tang J, Bello F, Kneebone R, Dasgupta P, Jaye P (2012) Validation and educational impact of distributed simulation in urology. *Journal of Endourology,* 26, A49.

Brindley PG, Reynolds SF (2011) Improving verbal communication in critical care medicine. *Journal of Critical Care,* 26(2), 155–159.

Brown JS, Collins A, Duguid P (1989) Situated cognition and the culture of learning. *Educational Researcher,* 18(1), 32–42.

Buck GH (1991) Development of simulators in medical education. *Gesnerus,* 48(1), 7–28.

Cao CG, Weinger MB, Slagle J et al. (2008) Differences in day and night shift clinical performance in anesthesiology. *Human Factors,* 50(2), 276–290.

Capella J, Smith S, Philp A et al. (2010) Teamwork training improves the clinical care of trauma patients. *Journal of Surgical Education,* 67(6), 439–443.

Cerrone SA, Adelman P, Akbar S, Yacht AC, Fornari A (2017) Using objective structured teaching encounters (OSTEs) to prepare chief residents to be emotionally intelligent leaders. *Medical Education Online,* 22(1), article 1320186.

Cheng A, Eppich W, Grant V, Sherbino J, Zendejas B, Cook DA (2014) Debriefing for technology-enhanced simulation: a systematic review and meta-analysis. *Medical Education,* 48, 657–666.

Cheng A, Kessler D, Mackinnon R et al. for the International Network for Simulation-based Pediatric Innovation, Research, and Education (INSPIRE) Reporting Guidelines Investigators (2016) Reporting guidelines for health care simulation research: extensions to the CONSORT and STROBE statements. *Advances in Simulation,* 1(25).

Clutterbuck D (2004) *Everyone Needs a Mentor: Fostering Talent in your Organisation.* London: CIPD Publishing.

Cohen D, Rhydderch M, Cooper I (2014) Managing remediation. In: Swanwick T (ed.) *Understanding Medical Education: Evidence, Theory and Practice,* 2nd edn. Chichester: Wiley-Blackwell.

Collins JP, Harden RM (1998) AMEE Medical Education Guide No. 13: Real patients, simulated patients and simulators in clinical examinations. *Medical Teacher,* 20(6), 508–521.

Cook DA, Hatala R. (2016) Validation of educational assessments: a primer for simulation and beyond. *Advances in Simulation,* 1(31).

Cooper JB, Taqueti VR (2004) A brief history of the development of mannequin simulators for clinical education and training. *Quality and Safety in Health Care,* 13, i11–i18.

CQHCA (Committee on Quality of Health Care in America) (1999) *To Err Is Human.* Washington, DC: National Academies Press.

Creswell J (2011) *Educational Research: Planning, Conducting, and Evaluating Quantitative and Qualitative Research,* 4th ed. Boston: Pearson.

Crookall D (2014) Engaging (in) gameplay and (in) debriefing. *Simulation and Gaming,* 45(4–5), 416–427.

Cruess RL, Cruess SR, Steinert Y (eds) (2009) *Teaching Medical Professionlism.* Cambridge: Cambridge University Press.

Davies S (2012) Embracing reflective practice. *Education for Primary Care,* 23, 9–12.

Dawe SR, Windsor JA, Broeders JA, Cregan PC, Hewett PJ, Maddern GJ (2014) A systematic review of surgical skills transfer after simulation-based training: laparoscopic cholecystectomy and endoscopy. *Annals of Surgery,* 259(2), 236–248.

Decker S, Fey M, Sideras S et al. (2013) Standards of best practice: Simulation Standard VI: The debriefing process. *Clinical Simulation in Nursing*, 9(6), e26–e29.

Dennick R (2012) Twelve tips for incorporating educational theory into teaching practices. *Medical Teacher*, 34(8), 618–624.

Dewey J (1933) *How We Think. A Restatement of the Relation of Reflective Thinking to the Educative Process*, revised edn. Boston: DC Heath.

Donaldson L (2008) *150 years of the Annual Report of the Chief Medical Officer*. http://webarchive.nationalarchives.gov.uk/+/http://www.dh.gov.uk/en/Publicationsandstatistics/Publications/AnnualReports/DH_096206 (accessed February 2019).

Dong Y, Harpreet SS, Cook DA et al. (2010) Simulation-based objective assessment discerns clinical proficiency in central line placement. *Chest*, 137, 1050–1056.

Draycott T, Sibanda T, Owen L et al. (2006) Does training in obstetric emergencies improve neonatal outcome? *British Journal of Obstetrics and Gynaecology*, 113(2), 177–182.

Dunning D, Heath C, Suls J (2004) Flawed self-assessment: implications for health, education, and the workplace. *Psychological Science in the Public Interest*, 5, 69–106.

Engestrom Y (2000) Activity theory as a framework for analyzing and redesigning work. *Ergonomics*, 43(7), 960–974.

Epstein RM (2007) Assessment in medical education. *New England Journal of Medicine*, 356, 387–396.

Ericsson KA (2004) Deliberate practice and the acquisition and maintenance of expert performance in medicine and related domains. *Academic Medicine*, 79(suppl 10), S70–S81.

Ericsson KA, Krampe RT, Tesch-Romer C (1993) The role of deliberate practice in the acquisition of expert performance. *Psychological Review*, 100(3), 363–406.

Eva KW, Armson H, Holmboe E, Lockyer J, Loney E, Mann K, Sargeant J (2012) Factors influencing responsiveness to feedback: on the interplay between fear, confidence and reasoning processes. *Advances in Health Sciences Education*, 17(1), 15–26.

Evans CJ, Harder N (2013) A formative approach to student remediation. *Nurse Educator*, 38 (4), 147–151.

Fanning RM, Gaba DM (2007) The role of debriefing in simulation-based learning. *Simulation in Healthcare*, 2(2), 115–125.

Fenwick T, Edwards R, Sawchuk P (2011) *Emerging Approaches to Educational Research: Tracing the Socio-Material*. London: Routledge.

Fletcher G, Flin R, McGeorge P, Glavin R, Maran N, Patey R (2003) Anaesthetists' non-technical skills (ANTS): evaluation of a behavioural marker system. *British Journal of Anaesthesia*, 90(5), 580–588.

Fletcher GCL, McGeorge P, Flin RH, Glavin RJ, Maran NJ (2002) The role of non-technical skills in anaesthesia: a review of current literature. *British Journal of Anaesthesia*, 88(3), 418–429.

Flin R, Winter J, Sarac C, Raduma M (2009) *Human Factors in Patient Safety: Review of Topics and Tools*. Geneva: World Health Organisation.

Forrest K, McKimm J, Edgar S (eds) (2013) *Essential Simulation in Clinical Education*. Chichester: Wiley Blackwell.

Frank JR, Snell SR, Ten Cate O et al. (2010) Competency-based medical education: theory to practice. *Medical Teacher*, 32, 638–645.

Gaba D (1992) Improving anesthesiologists performance by simulating. *Anesthesiology*, 76, 491–494.

Gaba D (2004) The future vision of simulation in health care. *Quality and Safety in Health Care*, 13, i2–i10.

Gaba D (2015) Expert's corner: research in healthcare simulation. In: Palaganas J, Maxworthy J, Epps C, Mancini M (eds) *Defining Excellence in Simulation Programs*. Philadelphia: Wolters Kluwer, p. 607.

Gaba D, Fish K, Howard S (1994) *Crisis Management in Anesthesiology*, 1st edn. Edinburgh: Churchill Livingston.

Gale TCE, Roberts MJ, Sice PJ et al. (2010) Predictive validity of a new selection centre testing non-technical skills for recruitment to training in anaesthesia. *British Journal of Anaesthesia*, 105(5), 603–609.

Gallagher AG, Cates CU (2004) Approval of virtual reality training for carotid stenting: what this means for procedural-based medicine. *JAMA*, 292(24), 3024–3026.

Gallagher AG, Neary P, Gillen P, Lane B, Whelan A, Tanner WA, Traynor O (2008) Novel method for assessment and selection of trainees for higher surgical training in general surgery. *ANZ Journal of Surgery*, 78(4), 282–290.

Garvey B, Garrett-Harris R (2005) *The Benefits of Mentoring: A Literature Review for East Mentor's Forum*. Sheffield: The Mentoring and Coaching Research Unit, Sheffield Hallam University.

Gillon R (1994) Medical ethics: four principles plus attention to scope. *British Medical Journal*, 309, 184–188.

GMC (General Medical Council) (2014) *Good Medical Practice*. London: General Medical Council.

GMC (General Medical Council) (2017) *Standards and Guidance for Postgraduate Curricula*. www.gmc-uk.org/education/postgraduate/standards_for_curricula.asp (accessed February 2019).

Goldstein RS (2005) Management of the critically ill patient in the emergency room: focus on safety issues. *Critical Care Clinician*, 21(1), 81–89, viii–ix.

Gottlieb R, Baechle MA, Janus C, Lanning SK (2017) Predicting performance in technical preclinical dental courses using advanced simulation. *Journal of Dental Education*, 81(1), 101–9.

Guba E (1981) Criteria for assessing the trustworthiness of naturalistic inquiries. *Educational Technology Research and Development*, 29 (2), 75–91.

Guise JM, Mladenovic J (2013) In situ simulation: identification of systems issues. *Seminars in Perinatology*, 37(3), 161–165.

Hamstra SJ, Brydges R, Hatala R, Zendejas B, Cook DA (2014). Reconsidering fidelity in simulation-based training. *Academic Medicine*, 89(3), 387–392.

Harden R, Stevenson M, Downie WW, Wilson GM (1975) Assessment of clinical competence using objective structured examination. *British Medical Journal*, 1(5955), 447–451.

Heron J (1986) *Six Category Intervention Analysis*. Guildford: Human Potential Research Project, University of Surrey.

Hertel JP, Millis BJ (2002) *Using Simulations to Promote Learning in Higher Education: An Introduction*. Sterling, VA: Stylus Publishing.

Hesketh EA, Laidlaw JM (2002) Developing the teaching instinct, 1: feedback. *Medical Teacher*, 24(3), 245–248.

Hewett DG, Watson BM, Gallois C, Ward M, Leggett BA (2009) Intergroup communication between hospital doctors: implications for quality of patient care. *Social Science and Medicine*, 69(12), 1732–1740.

Honey MLL, Diener S, Conner K, Veltman M, Bodily D (2009) Teaching in virtual space: *Second Life* simulation for haemorrhage management [interactive session]. In: *Proceedings ascilite 2009 Auckland*, pp. 1222–1224. http://citeseerx.ist.psu.edu/viewdoc/download?doi=10.1.1.411.7927&rep=rep1&type=pdf (accessed February 2019).

Horley R (2008) Simulation and skill centre design. In: Riley RH (ed.) *Manual of Simulation in Healthcare*. New York: Oxford University Press.

Huba ME, Freed JE (2000) *Learner-Centred Assessment on College Campuses: Shifting the Focus from Teaching to Learning*. Cambridge: Pearson.

Huddy JR, Weldon S-M, Ralhan S, Painter T, Hanna GB, Kneebone R, Bello F (2016) Sequential simulation (SqS) of clinical pathways: a tool for public and patient engagement in point-of-care diagnostics. *BMJ Open*, 6(9), e011043.

Imperial College London (2014) *The London Handbook for Debriefing*. London: Imperial College. Available at: https://emergencypedia. files.wordpress.com/2014/03/london-debrifing.pdf (accessed February 2019).

International Task Force on Assessment Center Guidelines (2009) Guidelines and ethical considerations for assessment center operations. *International Journal of Selection and Assessment*, 17(3), 243–253.

Issenberg BS, McGaghie WC, Petrusa ER, Lee Gordon D, Scalese RJ (2005) Features and uses of high-fidelity medical simulations that lead to effective learning: a BEME systematic review. *Medical Teacher*, 27(1), 10–28.

JISC (Joint Information Systems Committee) (2015) *Feedback and Feed Forward: Using Technology to Support Students' Preogression Over Time*. http://www.jisc.ac.uk/guides/feedback-and-feed-forward (accessed February 2019).

Kassab E, Kyaw Tun J, Arora S et al. (2011) 'Blowing up the barriers': exploring and validating a new approach to simulation. *Annals of Surgery*, 254(6), 1059–1065.

Kassab E, Kyaw Tun J, Kneebone R (2012) A novel approach to contextualised surgical simulation training. *Simulation in Healthcare*, 7(3), 155–161.

Ker S (2003) Developing professional skills for practice – the results of a feasibility study using a reflective approach to intimate examination. *Medical Education*, 37(suppl 1), 34–41.

Kilminster SM, Jolly BC (2000) Effective supervision in clinical practice settings: a literature review. *Medical Education*, 34(10), 827–840.

King HB, Battles J, Baker DP et al. (2008) TeamSTEPPS: team strategies and tools to enhance performance and patient safety. In: Henriksen K, Battles JB, Keyes MA, Grady ML (eds) *Advances in Patient Safety: New Directions and Alternative Approaches (Vol. 3: Performance and Tools)*. Rockville, MD: Agency for Healthcare Research and Quality.

Kirkpatrick DL (1994) *Evaluating Training Programmes: The Four Levels*. San Francisco: Berrett-Koehler.

Kneebone R (2009) Perspective: simulation and transformational change: the paradox of expertise. *Academic Medicine*, 84, 954–957.

Kneebone R (2010) Simulation, safety and surgery. *Quality and Safety in Health Care*, 19(suppl 3), 47–52.

Kneebone R (2015) When I say… reciprocal illumination. *Medical Education*, 49(9), 861–862.

Kneebone R, Arora S, King D et al. (2010) Distributed simulation – accessible immersive training. *Medical Teacher*, 32(1), 65–70.

Kneebone R, Kidd J, Nestel D, Asvall S, Paraskeva P, Darzi A (2002) An innovative model for teaching and learning clinical procedures. *Medical Education* 36, 628–634.

Kneebone R, Weldon S-M, Bello F (2016) Engaging patients and clinicians through simulation: rebalancing the dynamics of care. *Advances in Simulation (London)*, 1, 19.

Kolb DA (1984) *Experiential Learning: Experience as the Source of Learning and Development*. Englewood Cliffs, NJ: Prentice Hall.

Kolb DA, Boyatzis RE, Mainemelis C (2001) Experiential learning theory: previous research and new directions. In: Sternberg RJ (ed.) *Perspectives on Thinking, Learning, and Cognitive Styles*. New York: Routledge.

Lederman LC (1992) Debriefing: toward a systematic assessment of theory and practice. *Simulation and Gaming*, 23(2), 145–160.

Lewis, K.L, Bohnert, CA, Gammon, WL et al. (2017) The Association of Standardized Patient Educators (ASPE) standards of best practice (SOBP). *Advances in Simulation*, 2(1), 10.

Livingston LL, West CA, Livingston JL, Landry KA, Watzak BC, Graham LL (2016) Simulated disaster day: benefit from lessons learned through years of transformation from silos to interprofessional education. *Simulation in Healthcare*, 11(4), 293–298.

Maignan M, Koch FX, Chaix J, et al. (2016) Team Emergency Assessment Measure (TEAM) for the assessment of non-technical skills during resuscitation: validation of the French version. *Resuscitation*, 101, 115–120.

Maloney S, Haines T (2016) Issues of cost-benefit and cost-effectiveness for simulation in health professions education. *Advances in Simulation*, 1(13).

Maran N, Glavin R (2003) Low-to-high-fidelity simulation – a continuum of medical education? *Medical Education*, 37(suppl 1), 22–28.

Martin F (2016) *Developing Standardized Guidelines for Simulation Based Research*. http://blogs.biomedcentral.com/on-medicine/2016/09/01/developing-standardized-guidelines-simulation-based-research (accessed February 2019).

Mazzocco K, Petitti DB, Fong KT et al. (2009) Surgical team behaviors and patient outcomes. *American Journal of Surgery*, 197(5), 678–685.

McGaghie WC (2010) Medical education research as translational science. *Science Translational Medicine*, 19(2), 19cm8.

McGaghie WC, Draycott TJ, Dunn WF, Lopez CM, Stefanidis D (2011a) Evaluating the impact of simulation on translational patient outcomes. *Simulation in Healthcare*, 6 (suppl), S42–47.

McGaghie WC, Issenberg SB, Barsuk JH, Wayne DB (2014) A critical review of simulation-based mastery learning with translational outcomes. *Medical Education*, 48 (4), 375–385.

McGaghie WC, Issenberg SB, Cohen ER, Barsuk JH, Wayne DB (2011b) Does simulation-based medical education with deliberate practice yield better results than traditional clinical education? A meta-analytic comparative review of the evidence. *Academic Medicine*, 86(6), 706–711.

McGaghie WC, Issenberg SB, Petrusa ER, Scalese RJ (2010) A critical review of simulation-based medical education research: 2003–2009. *Medical Education*, 44, 50–63.

McGaghie WC, Siddall VJ, Mazmanian PE, Myers J (2009) Lessons for continuing medical education from simulation research in undergraduate and graduate medical education: effectiveness of continuing medical education: American College of Chest Physicians Evidence-based Educational Guidelines. *Chest*, 135(suppl 3), 62s–68s.

McGrath JL, Taekman JM, Dev P et al. (2018) Using virtual reality simulation environments to assess competence for emergency medicine learners. *Academic Emergency Medicine*, 25(2), 186–195.

McKimm J, Forrest K, Thistlethwaite J (eds) (2017) *Medical Education at a Glance*. Chichester: Wiley-Blackwell.

McNaughton N, Tiberius R, Hodges B (1999) Effects of portraying psychologically and emotionally complex standardized patient roles. *Teaching and Learning in Medicine*, 11(3), 135–141.

Miller GE (1990) The assessment of clinical skills/competence/performance. *Academic Medicine*, 65(9), S63–S67.

Mitchell G (2015) Psychology in education. In: Matheson D (ed.) *An Introduction to the Study of Education*, 4th edn. London: Routledge.

Nestel D, Brazil V, Hay M (2018) You can't put a value on that… Or can you? Economic evaluation in simulation-based medical education. *Medical Education*, 52(2), 139–141.

Nestel D, Cecchini M, Calandrini M et al. (2008) Real patient involvement in role development evaluating patient focused resources for clinical procedural skills. *Medical Teacher*, 30, 795–801.

Nestel D, Mobley B, Hunt EA, Eppich W (2014) Confederates in healthcare simulations: not as simple as it seems. *Clinical Simulation in Nursing*, 10(12), 611–616.

Nestel D, Muir E, Plant M, Kidd J, Thurlow S (2002) Modelling the lay expert for the first-year medical students: the actor-patient as teacher. *Medical Teacher*, 24, 562–564.

Nicklin J (2014) *My Trip to the Windy City*. SimGHOSTS 2014, USA conference. Unpublished.

Noeller TP, Smith MD, Holmes L, Cappaert M, Gross AJ, Cole-Kelly K, Rosen KR (2008) A theme-based hybrid simulation model to train and evaluate emergency medicine residents. *Academic Emergency Medicine*, 15(11), 1199–1206.

Østergaard D, Rosenberg J (2013) The evidence: what works, why and how? In: Forrest K, McKimm J, Edgar S (eds) *Essential Simulation in Clinical Education*. Chichester: Wiley Blackwell, pp. 26–42.

Papamitsiou Z, Economides A (2014) Learning analytics and educational data mining in practice: a systematic literature review of empirical evidence. *Educational Technology and Society*, 17(4), 49–64.

Patey R, Flin R, Fletcher G et al. (2005) Developing a taxonomy of anesthetists' nontechnical skills (ANTS). In: Henriksen K, Battles JB, Marks ES et al. (eds) *Advances in Patient Safety: From Research to Implementation (Vol. 4: Programs, Tools, and Products)*. Rockville, MD: Agency for Healthcare Research and Quality.

Pendleton D, Schofield T, Tate P, Havelock P (1984) *The Consultation: an Approach to Learning and Teaching*. Oxford: Oxford University Press.

Pickard S, Baraitser P, Rymer J, Piper J (2003) Can gynaecology teaching associates produce high quality effective training for medical students in the United Kingdom? *British Medical Journal*, 327, 1389–1392.

PMETB (Postgraduate Medical Education and Training Board (2007) *Developing and Maintaining an Assessment System – A PMETB Guide to Good Practice*. London: PMETB.

Posner G, Clark MD, Grant V (2017). Simulation in the clinical setting: towards a standard lexicon. *Advances in Simulation*, 2(15).

Powell P, Sorefan Z, Hamilton S, Sorefan Z, Kneebone R, Bello F (2016) Exploring the potential of sequential simulation. *Clinical Teacher*, 13(2), 112–118.

Pretz JE, Naples AJ, Sternberg RJ (2003) Recognizing, defining, and representing problems. In: Davidson JE, Sternberg RJ (eds) *The Psychology of Problem Solving*. Cambridge, MA: Harvard University Press, pp. 3–30.

Rajanbabu A, Drudi L, Lau S, Press JZ, Gotlieb WH (2014) Virtual reality surgical simulators – a prerequisite for robotic surgery. *Indian Journal of Surgical Oncology*, 5(2), 125–127.

Reason J (1990) *Human Error*, 1st edn. Cambridge: Cambridge University Press.

Regan L, Hexom B, Nazario S, Chinai SA, Visconti A, Sullivan C (2016) Remediation methods for milestones related to interpersonal and communication skills and professionalism. *Journal of Graduate Medical Education*, 8(1), 18–23.

Rehmann AJ, Mitman RD, Reynolds MC (1995) *A Handbook of Flight Simulation Fidelity Requirements for Human Factor Research*. Crew System Ergonomics Information Analysis Center, Wright-Patterson Air Force Base, Ohio.

Reid J, Stone K, Brown J et al. (2012) The Simulation Team Assessment Tool (STAT): development, reliability and validation. *Resuscitation*, 83(7), 879–886.

Rencic J, Durning SJ, Holmboe E, Gruppen LD (2016) Understanding the assessment of clinical reasoning. In: Wimmers PF, Mentowski M (eds) *Assessing Competence in Professional Performance Across Disciplines and Professions*. Cham, Switzerland: Springer International Publishing, pp. 209–235.

Riley RH, Grauze AM, Chinnery C, Horely RA, Trewhella NH (2003) Three years of CASMS: the world's busiest medical simulation centre. *Medical Journal of Australia*, 179, 626–630.

Roberts D, Roberts NJ (2014) Maximising sensory learning through immersive education. *Journal of Nursing Education and Practice*, 4(10), 74–79.

Rosen MA, Hunt EA, Pronovost PJ, Federowicz MA, Weaver SJ (2012) In situ simulation in continuing education for the health care professions: a systematic review. *Journal of Continuing Education in the Health Professions*, 32(4), 243–254.

Ross K (2012) Practice makes perfect. Planning considerations for medical simulation centers. *Health Facilities Management*, 25(11), 23–28.

Rudolph JW, Raemer DB, Simon R (2014) Establishing a safe container for learning in simulation: the role of the presimulation briefing. *Simulation in Healthcare*, 9(6), 339–349.

Rudolph JW, Simon R, Raemer DB (2007) Which reality matters? Questions on the path to high engagement in healthcare simulation. *Simulation in Healthcare*, 2(3), 161–163.

Salas E, Sims D, Burke C (2005) Is there a "big five" in teamwork? *Small Group Research*, 36(5), 555–599.

Sawyer T, Eppich W, Brett-Fleegler M et al. (2016) More than one way to debrief: a critical review of healthcare simulation debriefing methods. *Simulation in Healthcare* 11(3), 209–217.

Schmidt RA (1991) Frequent augmented feedback can degrade learning: evidence and interpretations. In: Stelmach GE, Requin J (eds) *Tutorials in Motor Neuroscience*. Dordrecht: Kluwer, pp. 59–76.

Sevdalis N, Nestel D, Kardong-Edgren S, Gaba DM (2016) A joint leap into a future of high-quality simulation research – standardizing the reporting of simulation science. *Advances in Simulation*, 1(24).

Shenton A (2004) Strategies for ensuring trustworthiness in qualitative research projects. *Education for Information*, 22, 63–75.

Silverman JD, Kurtz SM, Draper J (1996) The Calgary-Cambridge approach to communication skills teaching 1: Agenda-led, outcome-based analysis of the consultation. *Journal of Education in General Practice*, 7, 288–299.

SIRC (Simulation Innovation Resource Center) (2019) Glossary. https://sirc.nln.org/mod/glossary/print.php?id=183&mode=letter&hook=S&sortkey=&sortorder=&offset=-10 (accessed February 2019).

Skinner BF (1963) *Science and Human Behavior*. New York: Appleton.

Snow R (2014) Real patient participation in simulations. In: Nestel D, Bearman M (eds) *Simulated Patient Methodology: Theory, Evidence and Practice*. Oxford: Wiley-Blackwell.

St Pierre M, Hofinger G, Buerschaper C (2008) *Crisis Management in Acute Care Settings: Human Factors and Team Psychology in a High-Stakes Environment*. New York: Springer.

Stirling K, Hogg, G, Ker J, Anderson F, Hanslip J, Byrne D (2012) Using simulation to support doctors in difficulty. *Clinical Teacher*, 9, 285–289. doi: 10.1111/j.1743-498X.2012.00541.x.

Sunderland AB, Mackenzie R, Aldridge M (2014) *Faculty Development for Simulation-Based Education: A Systematic Review*. Unpublished.

Tribe HC, Harris A, Kneebone R (2018) Life on a knife edge: using simulation to engage young people in issues surrounding knife crime. *Advances in Simulation (London)*, 3, 20.

Tun JK, Granados A, Mavroveli S, Nuttall S, Brown R, Bello F, Kneebone R (2012) Simulating various levels of clinical challenge in the assessment of clinical procedure competence. *Annals of Emergency Medicine*, 60(1), 112–120.

van der Ridder JMM, Stokking KM, McGaghie WC, ten Cate OTJ (2008) What is feedback in clinical education? *Medical Education*, 42, 189–197.

Varkey P, Gupta P, Arnold JJ, Torsher LC (2009) An innovative team collaboration assessment tool for a quality improvement curriculum. *American Journal of Medical Quality*, 24(1), 6–11.

Vygotsky LS (1978) *Mind in Society: The Development of Higher Psychological Processes*. Cambridge, MA: Harvard University Press.

Vygotsky LS (2003) *Psicologia pedagógica*. Porto Alegre, RS: Artmed. (Original work published 1926.)

Walsh K (2005) The rules. *British Medical Journal*, 331(7516), 574.

Weaver SJ, Dy SM, Rosen MA (2014) Team-training in healthcare: a narrative synthesis of the literature. *BMJ Quality and Safety*, 23(5), 359–372.

Weil A, Weldon SM, Kronfli M, Watkins B, Kneebone R, Bello F, Cox S (2018) A new approach to multi-professional end of life care training using a sequential simulation (SqS Simulation™) design: a mixed methods study. *Nurse Education Today*, 71, 26–33.

Weldon S-M, Coates L, Kneebone R, Bello F (2015b) Hounslow whole system integrated model of care sequential simulation (SqS) workshops, Health Education North West London – simulation: is a new approach needed? HEE NWL Simulation Conference, conference paper.

Weldon S-M, Kneebone R, Bello F (2016) Collaborative healthcare remodelling through sequential simulation: a patient and front-line staff perspective. *BMJ Simulation and Technology Enhanced Learning*, 2, 78–86.

Weldon S-M, Ralhan S, Paice E, Kneebone R, Bello F (2015a) Sequential simulation (SqS): an innovative approach to educating GP receptionists about integrated care via a patient journey – a mixed methods approach. *BMC Family Practice*, 16, 109.

Weller J, Frengley R, Torrie J et al. (2011) Evaluation of an instrument to measure teamwork in multidisciplinary critical care teams. *BMJ Quality and Safety*, 20, 216–222.

Weller JM, Nestrel D, Marshall SD, Brooks PM, Conn JJ (2012) Simulation in clinical teaching and learning. *Medical Journal of Australia*, 196 (9), 594.

Whitmore J (2009) *Coaching for Performance*, 4th edn. London: Nicholas Brealey Publishing.

Wilkinson T (2014) Professionalism as the electricity of medicine. *Clinical Teacher*, 11(6), 487–488.

Wilkinson TJ, Wade WB, Knock LD (2009) A blueprint to assess professionalism: results of a systematic review. *Academic Medicine*, 84(5), 551–558.

World Alliance for Patient Safety (2008) *WHO Surgical Safety Checklist and Implementation Manual*. Geneva: World Health Organisation. http://www.who.int/patientsafety/safesurgery/ss_checklist/en (accessed February 2019).

Yardley S, Irvine AW, Lefroy J (2013) Minding the gap between communication skills simulation and authentic experience. *Medical Education*, 47(5), 495–510.

Ziv A, Rubin O, Moshinsky A, Gafni N et al. (2008) MOR: a simulation-based assessment centre for evaluating the personal and interpersonal qualities of medical school candidates. *Medical Education*, 42, 991–998.

Index

Page numbers in *italics* refer to illustrations or tables

Healthcare Simulation at a Glance. First Edition. Kirsty Forrest and Judy McKimm. © 2019 John Wiley & Sons, Ltd.
Published 2019 by John Wiley & Sons, Ltd.